Sharing my bedroom with a rabid dog; delivering twin foals and twin calves; fracture repair on an alligator; saving the life of a dog who loves her owner more than he loves her; surgery to remove an unexpected foreign object; assisting in human surgery; C-section on a cow in the middle of a pasture, etc., etc.

These are just a few experiences that contributed to the fascination, challenge and satisfaction in my life as a practicing veterinarian.

This book is for those interested in animals and their medical issues and how veterinarians deal with them. It is also about how rabies, one of the world's most dreaded diseases, played a very positive role in my practice in the early years. Anyone who is interested in pursuing a career in veterinary medicine may find it an interesting and perhaps motivational read that might give them an idea of what the next forty, fifty or sixty years of their life will be like.

Rabies Positive

An Animal Doctor's Memoirs

JERRY L. SIMMONS, DVM, MS

ISBN: 9798716918481 (paperback)

Table of Contents

Introduction

I have many stories to tell about experiences that I have had during my fifty year career in the practice of veterinary medicine. Memory fades with time but I have, as factually as possible, attempted to put those experiences into words. I regret that I'm not a "wordsmith" but I try to make up for that deficiency with true stories that give the reader interesting and enlightening insight into the veterinary medical profession. I have omitted the names of many of the people I write about. Frankly, I do not remember most of their names nor do I remember specific dates. But, most importantly, I do remember the experiences.

As a kid growing up in the small, north central Texas town of Keller about halfway between Ft. Worth and Denton I spent as much time as I could around cattle, horses, dogs and even a few cats. I was a member of 4-H, FFA and for a few years I was a young aspiring wannabe professional calf roper. I loved riding and could be found on a horse throwing a rope every chance I got. At sixteen years of age, while riding my favorite mare Polly on wet ground, she slipped and fell flat on her left side, breaking my left tibia. The fracture required a surgical repair and about six months on crutches which limited my ability to participate in high school sports that I enjoyed but did not dampen my love for horses and riding. As soon as I got my doctor's okay I was back on Polly throwing a rope at anything that I could imagine was a calf.

Whenever my dad's cows or horses needed veterinary care he would always call for one of the doctors at the Haltom City Animal Hospital which was located on the north edge of Ft Worth about fifteen miles from Keller. Fortunately for me, either Dr. Anderson or Dr. Heaton, two of the best and busiest large animal veterinarians in north central Texas, would make the call to my dad's place. I could not have hand-picked a better role model than either of them. I still remember how professionally they conducted themselves as they worked with the cattle and horses. While working outside on hot, muggy days I remember the white shirt and tie they often wore under their coveralls. They were, by any measure, honest to goodness profession-als. It was fascinating to watch them work and those opportunities, no doubt, planted the seed that would eventually grow into my becoming a veterinarian. As if being one of the best large animal doctors in the state of Texas was not enough, Dr. Anderson became the President of the Texas Veterinary Medical Association and then he served a term as the President of the American Veterinary Medical Association. I will always feel an obligation to him and Dr. Heaton.

While in high school I developed a desire to learn more about veterinary medicine and perhaps some day be like my role models mentioned above, so I applied for and got a part-time job at the Haltom City Animal Hospital working weekends, holidays or whenever I had a day off from school. Initially, I was a "cleaner". I cleaned just about everything in sight including but not limited to stalls, outside exercise pens and runs, small animal exam and surgery rooms, kennels, cages, large animal practice vehicles and anything else that looked like it needed attention. After a while the doctors asked me to assist with some of the small animal work and eventually I was asked to go on an occasional large animal farm or ranch call to help in any way that I could. I was an all around gofer but after time and a little more experience the doctors let me get more involved in the medical aspect of the work. This was invaluable "hands-on" experience that gave me a great deal of insight into the practice of veterinary medicine and unknown to me at the time would, a few years later, help me get accepted into vet school. Beyond all of that I actually got paid to work with animals and people I enjoyed being around in an environment in which I was comfortable. That job was possibly my first exposure to the concept of a positive correlation between work and compensation (both financial and psychological). I loved the work and, amazingly, I got paid for it.

I was in my second semester at North Texas State College in Denton, Texas, when I began to think seriously about how I was going to spend the rest of my life. I already had one semester of basic courses, including biology, and was well into my second semester, also including biology. Those were easily my favorite courses and my decision to pursue a career in a life science, especially one that involved animals, was an easy one. Veterinary medicine was the logical choice.

North Texas State did not have any animal science courses and I would not be able to finish the required pre-vet curriculum there. The only vet school in the state of Texas was at Texas A&M College and being a resident of Texas it would probably give me the best chance for admission (at the time I believe there were only eight or nine vet schools in the entire country). I finished the spring semester at North Texas State and transferred to A&M and entered the pre-veterinary curriculum the fall semester of 1960. I was accepted into the School of Veterinary Medicine the fall semester of 1962.

Traditionally, vet school requires four years of professional curriculum. However, because of a serious shortage of veterinarians at the time A&M changed to a three year, year-round curriculum starting with my class (Class of 1965). The advantage was that we would finish one year sooner and the disadvantages were that we were unable to work during the summer to help fund our schooling and most of us were completely exhausted physically and mentally by graduation. The school converted back to a four year program a few years later.

I graduated from the College of Veterinary Medicine on August 6, 1965, and returned home as soon as I could to begin my new job with Dr. Drew Ward at his small animal clinic in west Ft. Worth. I had been working in his clinic as an assistant for about a year, mainly on holidays or whenever I had a day or two off from school and had a way to get home from College Station which was about a three hour drive south of Ft. Worth. I received Texas license #2358 a couple weeks after returning home and immediately began the full-time job that Dr. Ward had offered me. My starting salary was $500 a month which was pretty good pay at the time for a new graduate. I had no other prospects for work and needed money sooner than later to support myself and start making payments on my school debt which was considerable. I got a lot of good experience during the short time that I was with Dr. Ward but his practice was limited to small animals (aka companion animal, primarily dogs and cats) and I wanted to do both small and large animal work (aka mixed practice). I was also considering limiting my practice to horses.

I decided that I wanted to do mixed or equine only practice and after about a month with Dr. Ward I said farewell to Ft Worth and hit the road looking for a another job. I interviewed at practices in Gainesville, Wichita Falls, Abilene and Midland. I couldn't help but notice how the farther west I traveled the more I liked the country, especially the drier climate and mountains that were beginning to come into view a little farther to the west. Eventually I ended up in El Paso which was as far west as I could go and still be in Texas which, at the time time, was the only state in which I was licensed, therefore the only state in which I could legally practice.

I arrived in El Paso at a time when rabies was rampant in the area. Ironically, as dreaded as the disease was and continues to be it contributed greatly to my financial survival during my early years in practice, which I will explain in greater detail later. It seemed only appropriate to recognize rabies contribution to my life and career by naming this book after it. The disease didn't "guarantee" my success but it provided enough workload to at least give me a chance succeed in a brand new start-up practice with almost no money and no reliable income stream that I could depend on. The only real assets I had were my DVM degree and a license to practice from the Texas State Board of Veterinary Medical Examiners. And then I had two less tangible assets but at least as important: desire and determination to make a go of it.

I thank the role models who motivated me to follow my dream, the teachers and professors who helped me achieve it and the mentors and colleagues who supported and encouraged me throughout my career. The many veterinary technicians, assistants and receptionists that I worked with were invaluable. My wife Edita who, in addition to being a homemaker and full-time mom for our three children, was the clinic office manager my entire career. Last, but certainly not least, I will forever be grateful to the thousands of clients who trusted me with the care of their animals.

I was fortunate to have spent my career practicing veterinary medicine during the profession's "Golden Age". My timing could not have been better. Much of today's technology which we might take for granted did not exist in the mid-1960's when I started practice. MRI, CT Scan, ultrasound, digital radiography and many other technical advances that are commonly used today in veterinary medicine were hardly heard of much less routinely used in private practice. Biologicals and pharmaceuticals have made huge technical advances since the mid-1960s. Practice today compared to that of fifty plus years ago is a good example of the proverbial apples and oranges: incomparable. It has truly been an exciting time to be a veterinarian.

After reading the Introduction one could easily believe that this book is an autobiography. Well, perhaps it is, technically, but only in the sense that it is about my life as "a practicing veterinarian". The experiences are what this book is about and they are not unique to my career. Any practitioner who has spent forty or fifty years of his or her life in the profession no doubt has many stories to tell about why it is so fascinating and gratifying and at times challenging, mentally, emotionally and physically. One who is interested in animals and their medical issues and how we in the profession deal with them, or perhaps is interested in pursuing a career in veterinary medicine, will find this book an interesting and perhaps motivational read. It is a good place to begin to learn about the profession and how, in the event that you do become a veterinarian, you might spend the next forty, fifty or sixty years of your life.

1

Search For Work

In my quest to find a job as a veterinarian in a mixed practice I eventually ended up in El Paso where I had never been and about which I knew almost nothing. The only person I was acquainted with in the entire area was Dr. Pinky Edwin, a vet school classmate of mine who went straight from school after graduation to El Paso to take over an established practice. I knew that there was a horse racing track on the New Mexico side of El Paso and another one in Juarez and that the two cities shared the United States/Mexico border. Other than that there were mountains and good snow skiing and a horse racing track (Ruidoso Downs) about three hours north in Ruidoso, New Mexico.

Sunland Park Racetrack is located on the western fringe of El Paso, near the Texas state line, but is physically in New Mexico. Sunland Park would hold races through the winter and when its meet ended most of the horses would be sent up to the mountains of Ruidoso to run at Ruidoso Downs until September. Then, after Labor Day, they would return to El Paso for the winter meet. So a vet could practice pretty much year round on the track and remain in the general El Paso/Ruidoso area.

My prospects for doing horse practice looked promising but I would need a New Mexico license and the next licensing exam administered by the State Board was about four months away. In the meantime, I needed work.

Shortly after arriving in El Paso, I visited Pinky at his practice and told him I was thinking about relocating to the area. He suggested that I contact Dr. Warren Nickerson, a large animal vet who was kind enough to take a full day out of his practice to show me around the El Paso area. Dr. Nickerson partnered with Dr. Claude Willey, also a large animal vet who was a member of the Texas State Board of Veterinary Medical Examiners at the time I took the licensing exam.

Dr. Nickerson gave me a tour of the greater El Paso area, from the upper valley to the lower valley. He introduced me to some of his cattle clients and showed me every small animal clinic in town. One of those clinics was The Animal Clinic on Alameda St. It was owned by Dr. Robert Butchofsky, who was looking for help in his practice. It was by far the largest mixed practice in El Paso and quite a few of the established vets in El Paso got their start with Dr. Bob. It was high-volume, predominantly small animal with considerable horse work and some cattle work. I told Dr. Bob that I intended to get on the race track as soon as I had a New Mexico license and that I needed work until the exam would be given again. He offered me the job starting at $650 a month, which was a substantial increase over the $500 a month that I made with Dr. Ward in Ft. Worth.

It was October, the best time of year in far west Texas. The area was beautiful and the people were friendly. I liked the mountains and the Rio Grande River and the high, dry desert climate. It was different from any place I'd ever been. As I recall the population of El Paso at the time was about 225,000. Ciudad Juarez, Mexico, just across the Rio Grande, and its cultural influence added to the intrigue. I loved the warm days and cool nights in the desert and I would get the large and small animal experience that I wanted and also have the option of eventually doing horse practice at Sunland Park and Ruidoso. All of this seemed to be everything I was looking for. It felt right so I accepted Dr. Butchofsky's job offer.

I drove back home the next day and announced to my parents that I had accepted a job in El Paso that appeared to be what I thought I wanted. And I would get a $150 a month raise. Although my parents would have preferred that I stay in the Dallas/Ft. Worth area, they were happy for me. After a couple days of goodbyes and loading my car with clothes and personal belongings, I was headed west again...back to far West Texas. Little did I have the slightest idea that fifty-five years later I would still be living here.

A monthly salary of $650 in the mid-1960's might not sound like much by today's standards, but at the time it was good pay for a recently graduated veterinarian. It helped that I was single and had no personal commitment to anyone other than myself. I did have substantial student loan commitments to Texas A&M and the Riverside State Bank in Fort Worth. Obviously, it would have been different if I'd had a family. In that case, I probably would have stayed in the Dallas/Fort Worth area. But, I was flexible and fairly certain that I could live and make payments on my car and school loans on $650 a month.

My time at The Animal Clinic was a good experience. Dr. Butchofsky was an excellent practitioner on both small and large animals and I learned a lot from him. He paid me well but he also got his money's worth. Office hours were 8 am to 6 pm six days a week and 9 am to noon Sunday. We made large animal calls almost every day before and after regular clinic hours. 12 hour days were not uncommon and we routinely worked during lunch, grabbing a tamale or taco or enchilada between clients or surgeries. This was long before after hours and weekend emergency clinics came into being, so after hours trips back to the clinic or outside farm calls were common.

I got along well with the staff and especially enjoyed working with Pepe, a kennel worker who to this day is one of the funniest people I have ever known. I could speak no spanish and Pepe could speak very little english so he took it upon himself to teach me as much spanish as he could within a short time. Thanks to Pepe when I left four months later I had a pretty good working knowledge of espanol that was at best marginally proper.

I stayed in cheap motels for the first couple of weeks after starting work for Dr. Butchofsky. Since I worked seven days a week all I really needed was a place to shower and sleep. I met Bill Wilson, who worked for the Texas Alcohol Control Commission. He was looking to share an apartment that he rented on Pershing Drive in central El Paso. It was nothing fancy but adequate and the rent was affordable. We got along well and continued to be friends for several years until he was transferred back to Austin.

He knew a lot of horse owners and trainers at Sunland Park and gave me leads that were helpful when I started my own practice.

Dr. Bob didn't hold back on working me into his practice. He had long-time clients who would never think of going to another clinic or using another vet. I think his clients figured if I worked with Dr. Bob I must be okay. So I was thrown into the practice full-bore from the start. The high volume workload gave me a tremendous amount of invaluable hands-on experience. I loved what I was doing and work and long hours were never an issue.

I had few problems with small animal work because I always had access to either Dr. Bob or Joe, the head tech, for a quick consult. Large animal work was different since I would almost always be solo and I didn't carry a two-way radio (that was long before cell phones came on the scene). But I did carry two textbooks, one on equine medicine and surgery and another on bovine medicine and surgery. I was careful not to let the client see me refer to them in the middle of an exam or treatment. That's not exactly the way to instill confidence in a client. But a quick "look" while back at the car "to get an instrument or medication", as I would put it to the client, sure helped me a few times during my early years as a large animal practitioner.

2
On My Own

The New Mexico State Board of Veterinary Medicine licensing exam was held in Santa Fe on January 14, 1966, and I received license number 268. I was then good to work in New Mexico including Sunland Park Racetrack. I was tempted to start full-time on the track but doubted that I would be able to keep busy enough to cover my expenses for some time, given that there were already several established equine docs, full-time on the track. I rode with Dr. Joe Miller, one of the racetrack vets, on his daily rounds a few times which gave me the opportunity to meet trainers and owners who might eventually become prospective clients. I even thought about buying Dr. Miller's vacant clinic in Alamogordo, NM, but, as much as I liked the town and its close proximity to the Sacramento Mountains, I decided that I was already somewhat established in El Paso because of my association with Dr.

Butchofsky and could probably develop a practice here sooner than there. I never got a job offer from any of the regular track vets, but I never pursued that possibility either since they all seemed to be about as busy as they wanted to be. But then again, I was always fairly independent and never really thought much about working for anyone other than myself.

I decided that my best bet for success would be to start a general practice on the west side fairly close to the track, doing anything that I could find to do, with special emphasis on the track and off-track training facilities, of which there were several in the immediate area. There was a good equine population in the valley all the way up to Las Cruces, including hunters, jumpers, polo ponies and steer and calf roping horses. There were also a few small cattle feedlots and herds and a couple of dairies. The large animal prospects were promising, although what I didn't realize at the time was the excellent demographic make-up for small animal practice.

First order of business would be to establish an office which would be a point of contact for large animal clients and perhaps a small clinic for pets. After a couple days of searching I found a small adobe house only two blocks from considerable retail business at the Crossroads and about five miles from the racetrack. This would become my small animal clinic, large animal office and my residence, all for $100 per month. That was a lot of money at the time, especially for someone with no steady income, but its proximity to the track and its small animal practice potential, coupled with having a place to shower and sleep, all for $100 a month seemed like a pretty good deal.

My new clinic/residence was located on Conley Road, just off North Mesa Street and two blocks from Doniphan. It had about 1000 square feet of floor space with a living room, kitchen, bedroom, bath and a small closet in the bedroom. The living room would be my reception area, waiting room and business office. The kitchen behind would be my exam, treatment and surgery room. The kitchen cabinets would work for medication storage, the exam table would double as my surgery table and I could use the small refrigerator for vaccine storage and what little food I would be keeping. One wall separated the clinic from the bathroom and bedroom, which would also be my cage room for the one small portable cage that I owned. There was just enough space for a small bed in the corner of the room a few feet from the cage. The closet was small but would work for storage since my wardrobe was limited and required very little space. That's about it. It wasn't much but it was enough to give me a chance to hopefully get my career off the ground.

I was told by more than one person that there was no way I could develop a successful practice in this building and location but their "advice" only gave me more incentive to "make" it work. The building might have been less than optimal but the location could not have been better for a mixed practice and because of that I began to generate work and income almost from the day that I put up my sign in front of the house. I wasn't exactly swamped with work early on and there were many days when the phone never rang nor did a soul come through my front door, but there was still enough work to give me faith that I had made a good decision on location.

Turns out, this little casita served me well for about three years. It enabled me to follow a principle that is key to financial success: spend less than you make. Keep practice expense consistent with income, i.e., well below it. That wasn't difficult to do in that building. My operating expenses were extremely low and using the building as a residence helped immensely. It didn't hurt that I was also the receptionist, cage cleaner, bookkeeper and janitor and general all-around gofer. In retrospect, I think that if my monthly operating and living expense had been much more than $100, it's doubtful that I would have survived.

After a couple days of buying cheap furniture and settling into my new digs I began to make daily trips to the track to let the horse crowd know that I was around and available for work. I'd get there at daybreak and get coffee and maybe a little breakfast at the track cafe when I had enough cash. Then I would go to the stable area and cruise around to meet owners and trainers and let them know that I was looking for work. Little did I know that I would soon find work and at the same time be taught a cold, hard lesson about business and human behavior, a life lesson that I would never forget. As they say "I learn slow but I learn good", and what I learned from that experience would serve me well throughout my fifty plus year career, not only in practice but in other business ventures that I was later involved in.

There were many outstanding trainers and owners with stables full of top notch equine racers and the established vets already had them locked up. Being the newest vet on the track, I took what I could get, which, amazingly, was more than I had expected. Almost from my first day on the track I was busy: deworming, vaccinating, pre- and post-race exams, lameness exams and treatments and sick calls. But, there was a problem. I was so absorbed in my work that I failed to realize that I wasn't being paid. It became all too obvious that slow payment, or in some cases no payment, was rapidly depleting what little cash reserve that I had, making it difficult to impossible to keep current on my clinic rent and payments to my drug and supply vendors.

It was customary to bill either the owner or trainer for my services since working on a cash basis at the track was essentially not doable. Also, after the work was done and could not be undone, I was at the mercy of the client to pay me in a timely manner, which pretty much had to be within a month in order for me to pay my bills and eke out a living. Seldom did I receive payment that soon. Even for the clients who did pay, I would bill them twice a month and still routinely have to wait weeks if not a month or two to finally get paid and even then it was often only a partial payment and a promise for more soon, just enough to give me hope and continue to work for them and run up their charges even more.

After a couple months of slow to no pay from several clients who had run up big bills, I began to get it. I was working for deadbeats who every other vet on the track would not work for because they knew they were bad pay. I had a few horse clients who were good pay but most of those were off the track and there were not enough of them for me to survive. I was working for too many stables that had no money or no morals or simply no intention of ever paying me. They had a lot more experience with that kind of finance than I did.

After about two months I had big bills with my suppliers, some of whom were threatening to cut me off. A couple of them started shipping c.o.d., which did not help since I seldom had enough cash on hand to pay at the time of delivery. It was obvious that I would not be able to continue without more income. I decided that it would be best to swallow my pride after such a short career and leave the track to spend more time developing a general practice. I pleaded with my suppliers to trust me and give me more time. Two of them did and agreed to help me. Those were Jones Vet Supply in Denver and Miller Vet Supply in Ft. Worth. They carried me on their books for months with only an occasional token payment which was the best that I could do for a while. I was trying to show good faith and I knew that they were concerned but they never stopped shipping my orders. Eventually, I was able to get current with all of my suppliers, but I could not have survived without the patience and help that I got from Jones and Miller.

So much for my desire to have an exclusive equine practice. If I'd had more financial "staying power" I would eventually have been able to get better paying stables and make a go of it. But it was what it was and that staying power did not exist. I gave serious thought to moving back to Ft. Worth to get a job or possibly going back to work for Dr Butchofsky, assuming he was agreeable. But I liked El Paso and as frustrated and, at times, angry about my racetrack failure as I was, I never really seriously doubted that I could establish a successful practice here. There were plenty of other horses and some small herds of cattle between El Paso and Las Cruces and there certainly should be enough residential population to provide small animal work as well. I just had to make a new start and that would be in a general practice on El Paso's west side and Upper Valley.

3

Rabid Roommate

It was mid-summer, 1966, and I was leaving my clinic about seven in the evening after finishing paper work and tying up loose ends after a long day. I was tired but happy because it had been a fairly busy day, relatively speaking. As I walked to my truck a car pulled into my parking lot. The woman driver asked if the clinic was closed and I answered yes but asked what she needed. She then proceeded to tell me about an injured dog she had found on the side of the road that she thought had been hit by a car. She was not a regular client but I recognized her and remembered that I had treated one of her horses for colic when she was unable to get her regular vet. I told her to bring the dog on into the clinic and I'd take a look.

She and her teenage daughter, both wearing riding pants and high top English boots, were returning home after a day of riding at a stable near Anapra, NM, not far from Sunland

Park Race Track. While driving home they came upon the dog lying on the side of McNutt Road and both mother and daughter, being animal lovers, simply could not drive past an injured animal without stopping to try to help it.

Together they lifted the dog from the trunk of their car and carried it into my exam room and gently laid it on the exam table. I asked them to hold her on the table to be sure she didn't jump or fall off while I examined her. It was a shaggy, black young adult mixed breed female that I estimated weighed about twenty pounds. She did not have a collar or tag or any other identification, which made me suspect that she had been running with a pack of wild dogs that probably had crossed over the border from Mexico and had been roaming the desert just outside the El Paso west side city limits.

Anapra is a small town near the US and Mexican border in a desert area where wild animals freely cross the border without having to cross the Rio Grande River. There are dangers, however, such as the packs of wild dogs and coyotes that roam the area looking for a meal. The life expectancy of any dog travelling through the area was shortened considerably, especially if it was injured or weakened from malnutrition or disease and unable to keep up with the pack. If one of these was lucky enough to escape the cannibalistic predators, it then must negotiate the traffic on McNutt Road, which at times could be quite busy. It makes for a long, dry trip since about the only water a wild animal can freely access in that area is the river, which is about a quarter mile beyond McNutt and Anapra, and there is no guarantee that the river will actually have water, especially at certain times of the year due to nearby irrigation requirements.

As I began my examination I could see that the dog was disoriented, emaciated and unable to stand or walk. Her mammary glands looked as if she had recently been nursing pups. She was listless but quickly became agitated and would snap at any movement around her head. There was a slight separation between her upper and lower jaw as if she was unable to completely close her mouth. She was drooling and her face, neck and front legs were covered with mostly dried saliva. Those last three clinical signs really got my attention and I immediately put on a pair of exam gloves and a surgical face mask before I proceeded with my physical.

Her rectal temperature was 104, about two degrees above normal. There was no physical evidence of an injury which I would expect to find if she had been hit by a car. No lacerations, bruising or obvious broken bones. I was unable to get a good look at her mouth and throat because of her attempts to bite. She did show signs, however, that suggested she might have a neurologic condition, possibly systemic poisoning or an infection with inflammation affecting her central nervous system. The most striking, perhaps most telling, sign was her attempt to bite at any movement near her face.

I suddenly realized that I quickly needed to get mother and daughter away from the dog before one of them got bitten. I muzzled the dog and carried her to my bedroom, which doubled as my cage room, and put her in the one small portable cage that I owned. I doubted that she would live through the night.

I had never seen a case of rabies but had studied it in detail in vet school. I remembered well one of my public health classes where we were shown films of animals and people sick with the disease. One of them, in particular, was a young boy who was infected with rabies and died shortly after the video was made. It had such a powerful effect on me that fifty plus years later I can still picture him vividly. The videos of rabies infected dogs all showed pretty much the same signs as the one I had just examined.

The dog on my table showed classic signs of rabies, but the only way to definitively diagnose it would be by microscopic examination of the brain. I explained to the mother that I had a list of differential diagnoses, any of which might be responsible for the clinical signs, but rabies was at the top of the list until proven otherwise. Both mother and daughter were genuinely frightened by the prospect that they might have been exposed to a rabid animal. And being around horses as much as they were, both had scratches on their hands that could possibly facilitate the transmission of the rabies virus into their bodies.

There are ways that a practitioner can soften the emotional shock and fear that a client feels when told that her pet has a life-threatening condition or that she has been exposed to a life-threatening disease. That's part of the "art" of veterinary practice. But, I lacked experience with this type of situation and couldn't think of anything to say that would make these two people feel better. I explained the rabies quarantine, observation and testing procedure as they washed their hands and arms with an antiseptic soap. I felt badly for both, especially the girl, who because of this experience might never again be able to bond with an animal.

I told them that it would be a few days before I had a final diagnosis, but I would keep in touch with them. I also urged the mother to contact their family physician first thing the next morning and she assured me that she would. They both thanked me on their way out.

It was late and by then I had lost my appetite and was too tired to go looking for food, so I went to bed wondering how many people in the history of mankind have spent the night with a rabid dog in their bedroom, literally about four to five feet from their bed. I couldn't sleep. I spent the night thinking about the dog and the mother and daughter. When I wasn't thinking about them, I thought about how bizarre this experience was especially if, in fact, she did have rabies, one of the most dreaded diseases of all time, and I'm sharing sleeping quarters with her. In another way which some might consider bizarre, it was exciting to think that I might have actually witnessed and physically handled a case of rabies. I got out of bed several times to check on her. I spent the entire night listening to her breathing, which gradually became more shallow and rapid and began to have a gurgling sound due to the accumulation of saliva in her throat and lungs. Finally, at about five, the room went quiet. She died.

I had long since given up on sleep that night so I was up early, showered, dressed and ready for the day. I made a strong pot of coffee at five and had several cups while waiting until seven, when I knew Animal Control started answering their phone.

Straight up 8 A.M. the Animal Control truck pulled into my parking lot and backed up to the front door. After I filled out the necessary paperwork including the names and address of the mother and daughter and the history they had given to me, the officer loaded the dead animal into his truck and assured me that the head would be shipped to Austin that day and I would be notified as soon as the results were received. Shipping and testing would be expedited.

A few days later the results came by phone: positive for rabies.

My clients' physician, who called me the day after they were in my clinic to discuss the dog's clinical signs, agreed with my tentative diagnosis and had wisely already started the mother and daughter on anti-rabies treatment the day following their exposure. The mother and daughter had no problems with the rabies injections and all ended well.

I had carefully protected myself while handling her but could not be sure that I had not been physically exposed to her saliva. The possibility of an airborne transmission of the disease also concerned me, having shared my very small, poorly ventilated bedroom/cage room with the patient that night. So, I called City-County Health Department and spoke with a physician who recommended that I get a rabies vaccination followed by two more at a monthly interval. A month after the last shot I got a blood draw and was found to have a good protective level of immunity.

Word that a case of rabies had been diagnosed on El Paso's west side quickly spread and for several days I was swamped with people with their dogs and cats that were either past due on their annual rabies vaccination or had never been vaccinated. When my waiting room filled they would line up single file from my front door all the way out to Conley Road and on Saturdays we would work non-stop from 8 am to 6 pm, or until we had finally seen the last person in line regardless of the time. Of course everyone wanted their pets vaccinated for rabies and many also asked for other vaccinations that were not required by law but highly recommended, such as distemper, hepatitis, leptospirosis combination. We would also schedule routine surgeries and treatments, such as spays and neuters and dental cleaning, and my cursory examination of each animal would frequently reveal skin lesions, eye, ear and skin infections, dental issues and other conditions that needed to be more thoroughly evaluated by testing and appropriate treatment. In addition to the rabies vaccinations we would line up enough work to keep us busy for days at a time.

The local media, newspapers, television and radio would always do a wonderful job at getting the word out that a case of rabies had been diagnosed and pet owners would come running. City Animal Control officers would canvas neighborhoods and ask pet owners for proof of rabies vaccination. If the owner could not produce proof, the officer would give a citation requiring that the pet be vaccinated within a certain and short period of time, usually a day or two. I couldn't help but notice how many of the people who showed up with their pets had no idea that there was an animal clinic on Conley Road.

Rabies is one of the most feared and deadly diseases of man and animal (I mean for me personally, it's right up there with rattlesnake and spider bites!), but as bizarre as it might seem, it would ramp up my workload and generate income that I badly needed to pay bills, invariably a few of which would be past due. It was publicity that I did not have to pay for and income that I badly needed, and as a result I established many clients who stayed with me for the duration of my career.

4

Severe Reaction

It was 8 am as I was leaving an upper valley dairy where I had arrived about two hours earlier to treat a case of bloat in one of the dairy's top milk producers. She responded well and I was feeling pretty good about myself and my profession, but the rumbling in my gut reminded me that I hadn't eaten anything for about twelve hours. So, since I wasn't pressed to get back to my office soon, I swung by a small cafe about half way between El Paso and Las Cruces for breakfast and coffee. Before I could get out of my truck my two-way radio signaled a call. It was my receptionist, Mrs. Knowles, calling to tell me that a supervisor at El Paso Animal Control had left a message with my answering service at seven that morning. The supervisor didn't say why he called, only that it was urgent and asked me to call him as soon as possible. I told Mrs. Knowles to call and tell him that I was on my way back from a farm call and that I'd get in touch with him just as soon as I got to the office.

The supervisor was a no-nonsense guy who ran his department with military-like precision and had the respect of the local veterinarians that he dealt with every day. His department's most important function was to control the stray animal population in an attempt to also control or eliminate rabies. So whenever he called I always suspected that it would some- how be related to rabies.

These were anxious times for a young, in- experienced vet. It was 1966 and El Paso was in the middle of a rabies outbreak. Several cases of canine rabies and at least one case of equine rabies had been diagnosed over the last couple of months. I was always fearful of the worst case scenario, that I might misdiag- nose a case of rabies involving human expo- sure and be responsible for a human death. I thought about it every time that I would ex- amine a sick animal, especially if it showed signs that might even remotely be what one might expect to see with rabies. I tried to maintain perspective, but it required a lot of discipline. If I had any doubt about whether an animal had rabies, I would always refer it to Animal Control for quarantine or, if the animal had died, I would request that Animal Control ship its brain to Austin for testing by the state laboratory.

The incidence of rabies at that time was high and there were always several animals at the Animal Control facility that were being kept under quarantine. Any animal that showed clinical signs consistent with rabies infection, or if it had bitten a person, was required by law to be placed in quarantine for at least ten days, sometimes longer. If an animal had bitten a person and was taken to a veterinarian for examination, we were obligated to call animal control and report it as a bite case. Animal Control would then notify the bite victim's personal physician. If the animal had been vaccinated within the required time, which at that time was annually, Animal Control would sometimes allow it to be quarantined at home. But if there was no history of vaccination, it would always be quarantined at the Animal Control facility.

The local veterinarians each volunteered to examine the quarantine cases daily for one week at a time. It was his or her responsibility to observe and report any signs that might suggest rabies or any other illness. Each animal would be observed by a veterinarian on the first, fifth and tenth days of quarantine. If we saw anything suspicious that might possibly be symptomatic for rabies we would mark PRS (Possible Rabies Suspect) on the quarantine slip and sign and date it. The act of signing off on a PRS carried considerable responsibility and legal liability.

If a veterinarian marked PRS on the slip, a cascade of events would immediately be triggered, especially if a human bite case was involved. Animal Control would notify the primary referring veterinarian, the bite victim and the bite victim's physician. Almost always, the physician would start the patient on anti-rabies injections, the same day if possible. At the time the standard treatment protocol was for a daily injection of rabies vaccine for fourteen consecutive days. The injections were painful and would occasionally cause a serious reaction that would require hospitalization.

I called the supervisor as soon as I got back to my clinic. It was my week to do the daily exams and he wanted to talk with me about a bite case that I had checked a couple of days previously. It was a small, white, shaggy, one year old mixed breed female dog that Animal Control had picked up because she had bitten one of the family members and had no history of ever receiving a rabies vaccination. I remembered the case. On the day five observation she was much more aggressive than she was on day one. She refused to eat and when not being agitated would spend most of her time blankly staring into space. Those were not yet all of the classic signs of rabies but enough for me to justify marking it as a PRS.

The bite victim was a nine year old girl. Her doctor had started her on the anti-rabies treatment the same day that I marked it as a PRS. After her second or third injection, she almost immediately had an anaphylactic reaction and had to be taken to the hospital by ambulance where she was presently in intensive care. Her doctor called the supervisor and told him that he was hesitant to give the girl another injection. At the doctor's request the supervisor looked at the dog.

I asked him what he thought. He said that her owners told him that she had never been very friendly. Always a little snappy, especially with strangers. But they did say that it wasn't like her to bite one of her own family.

He said that she wasn't eating but many normal dogs refuse to eat while at Animal Control. He said that he thought that perhaps she was just fearful of being there and simply wanted to go home, but he did note that she became quite aggressive when he approached her cage.

He thought that it might be a little early to call this case a PRS. He asked me to go to

Animal Control that same day and rethink my tentative diagnosis, assuming that if I changed my mind the rabies treatment for the girl would be stopped. In other words, give the dog a few more days to show more positive signs of rabies and in the meantime retract the PRS. Understandably, he didn't want the city to be held responsible for the girl's sickness, especially if the dog did not have rabies. I remember thinking at the time that he and I had worked together on several cases and he had never questioned my judgement. This time I suspected that he was doing what he had been told to do by someone higher up the city's pay scale in order to protect the city in case things didn't go well for the bite victim, especially if the dog proved to be negative for rabies. I appreciated his position, but I had to do what I thought was best.

If ever a veterinarian has been involved in a serious public health predicament, I knew that was precisely what I was in. If that young girl continued with medical issues from the injections, or worse, I had better be right on with my tentative diagnosis.

I was met at the front door of the Animal Control center by the supervisor who then walked with me back to the quarantine area. The place was in an uproar, with what seemed like every dog barking at the top of its lungs. As we approached the suspect's cage, she was pacing from one side of her cage to the other in a wobbly gait. She was thin, almost emaciated. She had turned over her food and water bowls and they looked as if she had been chewing on them. She was weaker in her back legs than when I last saw her and her breathing was rapid and labored. She was the only dog in the immediate area that wasn't barking and she became aggressive at any movement in front of her cage.

As I moved closer to her cage she suddenly lunged at the cage door, aggressively trying to get to me. She looked confused, uncertain whether she should be attacking me or the cage door. She made a very unfamiliar sound that you would not expect from a normal dog. It was not a bark or a growl or even a cry. It was like a mixture of all three. In her rage, she chewed on the metal bars of the door for a few seconds, then she backed off and lunged at it again. After a few more attacks on the door she settled down somewhat. Then the supervisor moved closer to her cage to get a look and she lunged at him. He jumped back and I could see that his face was flushed. This time she left blood on the door and the saliva that she was drooling became mixed with bright red blood.

She had either broken a tooth or lacerated her gum but acted as if she was unaware of it. She showed no sign of pain.

There was something in her eyes that bothered me. It was a distant look, as if she saw me but looked right through me. She responded more to my movement than my presence. If I stood perfectly still she didn't seem to even know that I was there. But when I moved she would attack viciously.

I told the supervisor that I hadn't seen nearly as many cases of rabies as he had but that this didn't look like just a feisty little dog that wanted out of there. She was violent, more so than I considered to simply be a behavioral issue. I thought she was sick. No guarantee that it was rabies but it had to be at the top of the list of differential diagnoses. The only way to know for sure would be to send her brain to the state health lab in Austin. Of course, the main concern would be the child's well-being in the meantime.

I could see that he was having second thoughts about questioning my judgement. He said that the dog had only one more day to finish the ten day quarantine and that if she didn't die today he would euthanize her the next morning and get her brain to Austin by that evening. He would ask for stat testing and probably get the report back in a couple of days.

The girl's doctor asked him to call after I had seen the dog, but he thought it would be better if I talked with him and asked me to do so. I knew that I was on my own now. I had to decide whether to hold firm on my tentative diagnosis or back down. If I chose the former, serious, perhaps fatal consequences could result because of continuing treatment of the child. On the other hand, if I changed my mind and the treatment was stopped, the consequences could be just as bad if the dog proved to have rabies.

I badly needed to share this awesome responsibility with someone. The attending physician seemed a logical choice.

I called the physician while still at Animal Control. After describing the violent behavior and progression of clinical signs, I told him that I couldn't be absolutely sure that this was rabies. He asked me if I had ever seen a case of rabies. Fortunately, I could honestly answer yes, a couple. He said he hadn't, although he had seen a film in an infectious disease course in medical school in which a boy was in the latter stage of the disease. Curiously, that was probably the same film that I saw in a public health class in vet school. It seemed that back in those days vet students and medical students all saw that same film. It definitely made a lasting impression. No one ever forgot what they saw.

After telling me about the child's reaction to the treatment, he agreed that rabies was a possibility. He said that he would resume her injections that afternoon but would keep her in the hospital. I told him that I or someone from Animal Control would call him as soon as we got the lab report.

The dog died that night and the brain was shipped by bus to Austin early the next morning. A couple of days later the supervisor called to tell me that he just gotten the report: positive for rabies.

As badly as I felt for the girl, I cannot describe the relief that I felt when I heard the report. And perhaps a bit of pride, not because an animal had died of rabies or because a bite victim had a serious reaction to the rabies vaccine, but because I followed my instincts, relied on my education and had the discipline and will power to hold firm and ultimately make what proved to be the correct decision for the child and her family.

Being young and inexperienced, perhaps I could have changed my mind three or four days earlier, especially if the city had put more pressure on me. The signs were more equivocal at that time. But the progression of signs, especially what I saw on my last observation, could have been a chapter on rabies in an infectious disease textbook.

This incident was a major confidence builder for me. It was an experience that I would refer back to many times during my career for help in "judgement call" situations, of which there were so many.

It also changed the supervisor's attitude toward me from that of a "wet behind the ears" rookie to more of a "battle-hardened" veteran, which I wasn't yet but I was getting there fast. He said that from that point on he would do his job and let me do mine. I left that conversation with no less respect for him. Our friendship and good working relationship continued until he finally retired several years later.

The child finished her treatment while being confined to the intensive care unit at the hospital. Not long afterward she was once again a perfectly normal nine year old. The family doctor wisely chose to treat all members of the family and others who had recent direct contact with the dog.

5

Twins

I did quite a bit of obstetrics in cattle and horses early on in my career. I enjoyed it and needed whatever work I could get, but I never felt like the compensation was adequate for the time, effort and medications that I used. Market value dictated how much a cattleman could or would pay for my service. Market value was less a factor for horse owners but still was a consideration. Ob work in large animals almost always requires another person or two to help. Too often I'd be called out on a large animal call, ob or otherwise, and was told by the client that someone would definitely be there to help me with whatever I was there to do. I would arrive on time and the horse, cow or whatever the animal, would be loose in a several acre pasture or large pen with not another soul in sight. More often than not the patient was half wild, allowing me to get only within 10 or 15 feet before it would turn on its heels and run to the other end of the area. Usually, I would continue to pursue until I eventually caught the animal, but I would also kill a lot of time in the process. I could usually manage in most cases but obstetrics always required at least one helper which of course would increase my cost.

It was common for me to spend thirty minutes to an hour to finally catch the animal and then more time depending on what I needed to do. What should have been a twenty minute visit would turn into an hour and a half. When finished I would get back in my truck and find that my office had been trying to contact me to let me know that several small animal clients were waiting for me, "so hurry!"

By the time I would get back to the office, several of those would have given up and left. I couldn't blame them. It's not hard to understand why this became an economic issue for me just as it has for so many other young, aspiring mixed animal practitioners.

As a courtesy to the owner and because I was naive in thinking that I would be paid in a timely manner, I would almost always bill the large animal client and often wait for a month or two to be paid, if I was lucky. I finally figured out that perhaps a big reason why so often I would arrive at a large animal client's place only to find no one there was to evade having to help or "pay" me, or both. Small animal clients, on the other hand, usually paid in the clinic at the time the service was rendered. I knew little about the business of veterinary practice but it didn't take long for me to recognize the economic discrepancy between large animal and small animal practice. After a few years of mixed practice I figured that I was probably losing money when I was out in the field on a large animal call, taking a chance on not getting paid, rather than back at the clinic tending to small animals, knowing that it was almost guaranteed that I would.

Money aside, I enjoyed large animal practice which frankly was the main reason that I went to vet school. I particularly enjoyed the challenge of large animal obstetrics which usually involved my assisting in delivery of calves or, much less commonly foals, or an occasional prolapsed uterus. It was physically demanding and often time consuming but when cases went well it was gratifying. I had two ob cases, a mare and a cow, that involved twins, both within the first three weeks after leaving the racetrack and starting my new practice on Conley Road.

Twinning in cows is uncommon (about one in 200 pregnancies) and rare in mares (about one in ten thousand pregnancies) and as special as witnessing and participating in a twinning can be, sadly, more often than not the outcome is not good. Abortion of one of the fetuses is common and if one or both fetuses survive birth they often have health issues that will at least lower their value if not eventually cause their death.

The cow that I treated belonged to an upper valley farmer who had a small herd of Hereford cattle in a cow/calf operation. He called my clinic one day shortly after I had started my practice on Conley Road. As I recall, it was the first phone call that I had gotten that day and it was already mid-afternoon. The ring of the phone startled me and woke me up from a doze. I got my wits about me quickly and answered. Someone had told him about my being a new vet not very far away from his place and since his regular vet was not available he called me. He had a young first calf heifer that was in labor and had been for several hours. Her water had broken but still no calf. He asked if I would take a look at her. This was one of the first large animal calls that I had received and I was thrilled. It was all I could do to contain my excitement. I controlled my emotions and did my best to project a professional image on the phone.

His farm was in the New Mexico part of the

Upper Valley and would be about a twenty to thirty minute drive. I told him I'd be there as soon as I could. I gathered up all the medications and instruments that I thought I might need, turned the phone over to the answering service and headed north.

The owner was at the gate waiting for me when I arrived. He was tall and thin and I guessed he was in his sixties. He had the classic look of a farmer, tanned from many hours in the sun and wearing denim overalls and a sweat-stained straw hat. My first impression was a good one...I liked him. He thanked me for coming and explained that the cow had unintentionally been bred to a bull much larger than she was. She had been in hard labor for a few hours with no calf and now the intensity of the contractions was decreasing, which was what the owner was most concerned about. Fortunately, she was in a stall inside the barn. I drove through the gate and parked as close to the barn as I could. I couldn't help but notice how clean the barn and pens and corrals were and especially the small stall that the cow was in.

She was standing and turned around to look at me when I walked into her stall. I was impressed with how big her belly was and my first thought was she had one really big fetus that was either a breech (tail end first) or was hung up at its shoulder because it was too large to pass through the birth canal. The farmer had several buckets of warm water, soap and several clean towels all readily available.

Almost all of my difficult obstetrics cases were simply a matter of getting the fetus properly presented in the birth canal for a normal head first delivery. Seldom would I need the help of a puller if I could achieve proper presentation. A breech presentation, which thankfully wasn't common, was tail first in the canal and usually much more difficult. But most cases of dystocia (difficult delivery) that I attended were caused by breech presentation or a large fetus.

Using antiseptic soap and warm water we got her as clean as we could given the work environment. I put on an ob sleeve, lubricated it and entered the birth canal. Thankfully it was not a breech but the head of the fetus was doubled back making it impossible to pass. With a bit of manipulation I was able to straighten the neck and get the head and front legs into the birth canal. A few tugs on the front legs and a newborn calf was delivered. At first glance it appeared to be in good health although I was surprised that it was not larger. As the farmer cleaned and tended to the calf I went out to my car and got medication for the mother. I was met by the owner as I walked back into the barn. He excitedly told me there appeared to be something protruding from the birth canal that looked odd.

Odd it was. It was another fetus in normal presentation and ready to be delivered. I hardly had to do anything to help. I don't know who was more excited, the farmer or myself. This was my first ob case involving twins and it was pretty cool to be involved in spite of the adverse health issues associated with twins.

Both newborns appeared to be smaller than normal but in good health, at least for the moment, but after I explained the negatives associated with twinning, understandably the farmer's excitement was noticeably dampened. Twinning often results in abortion, calves that are considerably smaller and weaker and if a one of the calves is a female and the other a male, the female will be sterile and unable to reproduce.

After I finished my work on the cow and calves and was getting in my car to leave the farmer, with a checkbook in hand, asked me how much he owed me. I told him I would send a bill but he insisted on paying me. I needed the money and didn't argue. I left his place in a state of euphoria, certain that I had done a good job and gained a new client.

Within days of the cow twinning, I was called to the upper valley to check on a mare that was in labor. The owner was a local attorney whose regular vet was not available. The case was similar to that of the cow, except that the mare was lying on her side and was having mild, infrequent contractions. Word had spread in the neighborhood that she was giving birth and the news had drawn a crowd of observers, unfortunately. Mares in the process of delivering a foal are much more sensitive to their environment than cows. They are more likely to have a difficult delivery when strangers are hovering and talking. I told the owner that the crowd of people might be part of the reason that she was struggling to deliver and it would be good if he could ask them to leave. He did the best he could without taking a chance on offending some of his neighbors and friends. So most left but a few stayed.

She had been in labor for several hours but except for being somewhat fatigued she appeared to be in good health. After cleaning her with antiseptic soap and putting on an ob sleeve, I entered the birth canal. The fetus felt small, in fact smaller than one would expect, and its head was in normal presentation. The front legs had not yet entered the birth canal and with a bit of manipulation I was able to get them into normal presentation. A few tugs on the front legs and out came a newborn foal. I was surprised how small it was. After cleaning its nose to be sure that it was breathing, I reentered the birth canal with the intention of checking for lacerations or pieces of retained placenta. I almost could not believe what I found, it was the head of another foal already in the birth canal and thankfully in normal presentation.

Twinning in mares is rare which made this experience even more exciting for me. Both foals were quite small which is to be expected of twins. In fact, the combined size of the twins was about that of a single normal foal.

I advised the owner of the rarity of the experience and the negative health considerations of the twins, including death at or shortly after birth. He politely asked if it would be okay with me if he called his regular vet to look at the mare and foals the following day when he would again be available. I assured him that I had no problem with that at all. Sorry to say, I did not followup on this case knowing that his regular vet would be attending. But typically the outcome is not good and there was no reason to believe that this case would be different.

Even though I was struggling financially these two twinning experiences gave me faith that I was doing the right thing. I was certain that if I stayed the course, my workload would pick up soon, and it did.

I got a call from an upper valley cattleman regarding a young cow that was in active labor and having hard contractions with no results. Her water had broken but so far no delivery of calf. He asked if I was available and I explained to him that I still had a couple of small animals in the office for routine exams and I couldn't leave before finishing them, but that I should be able to get there within an hour or so. I asked him where she was, hoping that he would say that she was in a nice clean barn or shelter of some kind. That wasn't the answer that I got. She was in the middle of a pasture not even close to a barn. She was standing but he was unable to make her walk to move her into a shelter and he was afraid to try to load her into a trailer for fear that he might injure her or the calf. I told him to leave her alone until I got there. I suspected that this was not going to be an easy job.

I arrived at his ranch at about dark and he and his helper were waiting for me. Fortunately, I was able to drive my practice truck directly to the cow. She had been in labor for some time and was exhausted to the point that she didn't want to move. We could have forced the issue but I agreed with the rancher that there simply was no way to move her without almost certainly causing harm to not only her but the calf as well. Whatever I was going to do, I was going to do where she was even though it was far from optimal.

She was a first calf Angus heifer, of considerable value according to the rancher, and had been bred to a large Angus bull. She was small and it was obvious that the fetus was too large for the birth canal. It had a good strong, regular heartbeat and, fortunately, the rancher had not tried to deliver using a calf-puller. The mother cow had stopped having contractions and the uterus was flaccid.

I explained to the rancher that we had no choice but to perform a C-section in order to save the fetus and probably the cow as well. This was certainly not an optimal environment for any kind of surgery, but especially open abdominal surgery. There was no way we would be sterile. Clean was the best that we could hope for. After explaining to the rancher all of the possible post-op complications, he agreed to proceed with the surgery.

The first obstacle was lack of light on the surgical site which would be her left side flank area. Obviously I had to be able to see what I was doing inside her abdomen. The rancher sent his helper to the barn for the tractor which he drove back and after getting it properly positioned, we were able to get its headlights pointed at the surgical site. He then went back to the barn and brought back a couple of hand-held flashlights to give me a little better lighting inside the abdomen.

Since we had no source of electricity I would not be able to use electric clippers to remove hair from the surgical site. I did the best that I could using curved scissors. Then I scrubbed the surgical site several times using antiseptic soap and warm water. After thoroughly rinsing and drying, I applied another antiseptic solution to the incision site which would be about eighteen to twenty inches long. I numbed the incision site with a local anesthetic and then applied more antiseptic solution. I felt that I had a clean, but far from sterile, surgical site. Once I had the surgical drapes in place, I began the procedure.

Once inside the abdomen I quickly found the uterus with the fetus in it and partially elevated it through the abdominal wall incision. An incision into the wall of the uterus revealed an active fetus ready to get the heck out of there. I delivered the calf onto clean towels that the rancher and helper had waiting. They immediately went to work drying it, especially its nose and mouth, and massaging and stimulating it to breathe. It looked to be in good shape and soon began to breath.

From the initial skin incision to the removal of the calf from the uterus took only a few minutes. The uterus and abdominal wall incision closures required much longer but were routine. The only resistance she gave was when I injected the local anesthetic. Otherwise, she remained still and quiet throughout the rest of the procedure. I inserted a couple antibiotic boluses into the uterus and gave injections of antibiotic and oxytocin to contract the uterus and help clean it and control bleeding. The cow appeared to be in good shape and after a couple liters of intravenous fluids we were able to get her to stand. She began to pay attention to the calf and we were able to get her to walk to the barn by carrying her calf. She was exhausted but she followed us.

All in all it was pretty routine and I had done what I considered to be as good a job as possible given the conditions that I had to work in. I left three syringes of antibiotic with the rancher with instructions to give her one daily until finished. I returned the following day to check on her. She was up and around, eating and caring for her calf. Her temperature was normal. After a couple more days she developed a low-grade infection in the lower end of the incision. I instructed the rancher to continue the daily antibiotic injection until it was finished and showed him how to clean and apply antiseptic solution to the area once daily for a few days. She healed well and I removed the skin sutures after a couple weeks.

All in all this is just another example of how challenging but gratifying the practice of veterinary medicine can be.

6

Los Lagartos

In today's practice environment we seldom wait longer than overnight to get hematology and blood chemistry test results. Clinics with in-house blood testing equipment will have most results within twenty to thirty minutes. We receive pathology reports overnight and seldom wait for more than a couple days for those that require extended evaluation. Digital radiography will generate images immediately and, if we need another opinion, those images can be forwarded to a board certified radiologist and within minutes we get an interpretation from a specialist. Ultrasound studies can be performed in-house and diagnoses made in minutes. CT scan and MRI imaging, while not common place in private practices, are available in many larger metropolitan areas with board certified specialists available for interpretation. Those are just a few of the many technological advances that have evolved over the last fifty or sixty years that have vastly improved the quality of veterinary medical practice.

Veterinary practice was different in the 1960's. El Paso was isolated and the nearest schools of veterinary medicine, Colorado State University and Texas A&M University, where specialized diagnostics and treatment were available, were each roughly 750 miles away. Generally blood and tissue specimens had to be shipped to labs by bus or air which required special preparation and packaging. Lab results would be sent back by phone or mail. Shipping and testing would usually require several days of wait time. If I was dealing with an acutely ill animal, which was often the case, by the time I had test results in hand, the patient would have either responded to my symptomatic treatment, or not. Lab results would often be after the fact. If I needed information immediately, I would often call the Vet School at Texas A&M or Colorado State and get a consult from a faculty clinician. They were usually right on with their diagnostic and treatment recommendations. This helped save many acutely sick patients and prevented a lot of frustration on my part.

Today's practitioner is much better equipped to establish a definitive diagnosis within a short time using technology that was not available when I started my practice. In vet school we were taught to question, listen (to both the patient and the client), look, touch, smell—in other words to rely more on our senses and subjective observations from the client—in order to make a diagnosis. It was not unusual that a diagnosis would consist of a list of "differential diagnoses". We would narrow the list as best we could based on history, signs and judgment decisions and then we would administer "symptomatic treatment" based on the clinical signs and other information that we considered most significant. We were, even with limited or no testing, successful with our treatment more often than not.

I would occasionally get a case that I felt simply could not wait several days for test results for definitive diagnosis and treatment. An example is an animal with a disease that might be transmissible to humans, otherwise known as a zoonosis. Obviously, the sooner such cases are diagnosed, the better, and the El Paso City-County Health Department Laboratory helped on several occasions by running blood tests for me, often on a stat basis.

I had many cases that required a biopsy to collect a tissue specimen which would then be examined microscopically, typically by a veterinary pathologist. But the nearest ones were at A&M or CSU, which again would involve several days of waiting for a diagnosis. But El Paso had several pathologists on the human side and, fortunately, two in particular who took a special interest in my cases. Drs. Hart and Frerichs, both MDs, helped me tremendously by examining tissue slides microscopically and evaluating diseased or cancerous conditions that typically only a pathologist would be qualified to interpret. They both seemed to enjoy the challenge of veterinary pathology and were often surprised at the similarity between human and animal tissue. In fact, Dr. Hart purchased several veterinary pathology textbooks to help him with my cases. They both did excellent work and always delivered results to me in a timely manner which made my work so much easier and helped me do a better job. I have always believed that pathologists, both medical and veterinary medical, are ultimately the "doctor's doctor" and I was very lucky to have them available when I needed them.

Another professional who helped me with cases that required a specific medication that was not always locally available and that I would not ordinarily keep in stock, usually because of high cost and short shelf life, was Mr. Brilliant, who was a pharmacist at a local drug store. Whenever I would get a case that required a medication that I did not have in stock and for which my patient could not wait several days to get from an out of town distributor, I would tell Mr. Brilliant what I needed and he would compound it for me, often having it ready for pick up the same day. It was a wonderful service, a stress reliever and also enabled me to practice better medicine.

I had a case that involved an older dog that was blind in both eyes because of a mature cataract in each. The owners were not financially able to take it to a vet school for surgery and there were no vets in the general area at the time who were qualified to do that kind of surgery. So, I called a friend who was a local human ophthalmologist and he agreed to come to my clinic and perform the cataract extraction. The surgery went well and, even though new lenses were not yet universally available to animal patients, simply removing the completely opaque lens would restore enough vision for the dog to function much better with limited vision, especially in an area that it was familiar with.

In the late 1960's and early 1970's there was little demand for veterinary care for exotic animals, at least in my practice. I would see an occasional ferret or hamster or maybe a gerbil, but that was about the extent of my exotic animal practice. That has changed dramatically over the last fifty years and veterinarians who do treat exotics today commonly see ferrets, pigs, rats, skunks, guinea pigs, snakes and birds, just to name a few. Some vets become board certified and specialize in exotic animal medicine. Exotics have their own diseases and medical conditions that require specific knowledge of diagnostics, treatments, medications, anesthetic protocols and surgical techniques when compared to a routine companion animal practice. Zoo practice, including lions, elephants, giraffes, rhinos, etc., is an obvious example of the need for advanced, specialized training when treating exotics.

Everyone knows El Paso is a desert town situated in the high, dry climate of the Chihuahuan Desert. That's a big reason why I moved here in 1965 and continue to live here: I love the arid desert climate, the altitude, the lushness of the desert vegetation and how it springs to life overnight after even a brief rain that might produce unnoticeable results in many parts of the world, the beauty (and harshness) of the cacti, yucca, ocotillo and other vegetation that can handle the heat and prosper with very little water.

But alligators in the Chihuahuan Desert?? Come on you've got to be kidding me. Gators don't like high, dry areas. They prefer low, wet areas. Well, fact is there were several that did reside in the heart of downtown El Paso and invariably the first two questions that come to mind are why and when. We can answer the "when" question but the answer to "why" is more elusive.

There are differing opinions regarding the few details that are available but most agree that in the late 1800's the city created a small park in the downtown area and eventually added a pond to accommodate several alligators. The pond was surrounded by a wall and several trees were planted and a gazebo was built in what would be called San Jacinto Plaza, or, La Plaza de los Lagartos. As many as seven or eight gators resided in the pool at one time and for many years were a popular attraction in the city. A few of the gators' names were Minnie, Oscar, Jack and Jill.

After several pranks and incidents of vandalism in the early sixties, the gators were moved to the El Paso zoo in 1965 for safer keeping. They were returned to the pond in 1972 only to be sent back to the zoo in 1974 when the pond was permanently removed.

The gators had their disagreements with occasional scuffles but seldom resulted in serious injury until one day a fight ensued between two adults that left one of them with a fractured humerus (the bone between the elbow and shoulder). Word spread quickly and the general consensus among the public and the city was to do whatever could be done, if anything, to repair it. I got a call from a supervisor at El Paso Animal Control. We discussed possible treatment options and agreed that the only viable option was internal fixation with a metal bone plate. Obviously, any kind of external fixation, i.e., a splint or cast would be useless. If the fracture was not repaired, my guess was that the city would euthanize it or it would be finished off by its brethren in the plaza. He asked if I would be willing to try to repair it. I felt obligated to at least try, with "try" being the key word. So, I was about to become a "wildlife veterinarian", a career option that I always thought would be interesting.

The next morning three men from animal control arrived at my clinic in a van. They opened the back doors and very carefully removed the alligator, whose mouth was securely taped shut, at least I hoped that it was. One man was on the head, another was midbody and the third was on the tail. It was all the man on the tail could do to not be thrown to the ground by the gator's thrashing. They brought him into the clinic and put him on my surgery table. I don't remember exactly how long he was but I do remember that he hung over the ends of the table by a foot or so. As I recall, the table was five feet long. At this point there were two men on the tail and it was all they could do to hang on to it. The gator's sheer strength was awesome.

I don't remember much of the details regarding anesthesia and monitoring of the procedure. Anesthetic agents and heart/respiratory monitors weren't nearly as sophisticated and accurate as they are now, especially for use in an animal as exotic as an alligator. I think we used an anesthetic agent called ketamine possibly mixed with another drug to induce anesthesia and then we switched over to an inhalant anesthetic via an endotracheal tube.

We weren't sure that the fracture was amenable to fixation because we had no radiograph. The only way that we would know for sure was to open the fracture site and visually examine it, which is what we did. There was a mild crushing effect with some small bone fragments at the fracture site but probably not enough to affect healing. Because of the curvature of the bone we had to bend and shape the metal plate to fit. We attached and anchored it with three screws above and three below the fracture line and got what we considered suitable alignment and fixation. We then closed the incision.

Up to that point things had gone well. Sadly, however, the alligator never recovered from the anesthesia. I believe that if the same procedure were done today, given the increased knowledge of cardiopulmonary physiology in these beasts, along with better monitoring equipment, not to mention improved anesthetic agents, it would have at least had a chance for full recovery. Even though the outcome was not good, I was satisfied that we had done the best we could given what we had to work with.

The general public has limited knowledge regarding how much education, time and expense are required to become a Doctor of Veterinary Medicine. Minimum requirements for application to the professional curriculum is three to four years of pre-veterinary curriculum in college including basic science and math courses as well as history, english and several semesters of chemistry and biology. Many applicants have a graduate degree (MS, PhD or other degree) as well. The typical vet school professional curriculum is four years after which many new graduates will remain at a teaching institution for an internship (usually one year) and a residency (usually three years or more, depending on the specialty) or go straight from vet school to graduate school for a MS, a PhD or other post-doctoral degree.

A client once asked me if vet school took longer than barber school. I started to laugh then realized that he was dead serious. Certainly I intend no disrespect to barbers, but yes, it does require considerably more time and expense. As I write this the average debt for a recent graduate from veterinary school is about $150,000.

"Wow, that's just like a real doctor!" I have heard this comment many times from adults and children while I was using a stethoscope to evaluate a patient's heart and lung sounds. Thus, the terms "Real Doctor", and "R.D.", were coined many years ago and are still facetiously used by veterinarians.

Once, while I was attending a weekend meeting at the Texas A&M vet school, I was given a pin-on button that about says it all: "REAL doctors treat more than one species".

Another issue for me has been the public's lack of knowledge regarding the various medical conditions that practicing veterinarians often deal with. Some examples are infectious diseases, many of which that are transmissible to people, diseases of the immune system, osteoarthritis, kidney and liver failure, heart conditions including arrhythmias, congestive heart failure, congenital abnormalities such as patent ductus arteriosus, heart valve dysfunctions, pancreatitis, Cushing's disease, diabetes often with ketoacidosis, pulmonary thromboembolism, hyper- and hypothyroidism and many different types of cancer, just to name a few. And then there are orthopedic conditions such as a torn cranial cruciate ligament (in people known as an anterior cruciate ligament) in the knee, joint luxations, intervertebral disc disease, hip dysplasia, fractures and neurological conditions, again just to name a few. And dentistry, behavioral conditions, etc., etc.

Also, veterinarians contribute to the health and well-being of people by diagnosing and treating, or otherwise removing, animals with diseases—some common and others not so—that may be transmissible to humans (zoonoses). Some examples are: rabies, anthrax, brucellosis, leptospirosis, pasteurellosis, ringworm, toxoplasmosis, mange, intestinal parasitic infestations and many more. Veterinarians who specialize in public health conditions such as these usually attend graduate school for advanced education and a graduate degree (MPh, PhD.)

My front desk would get a call almost daily from someone who would talk about how their dog or cat had a bump somewhere on its body, or she wouldn't eat her breakfast, or he threw up last night, or had diarrhea this morning, or, and this one is my favorite, he's just not acting right (a condition that we in the profession affectionately refer to as "ADR", aka, "Ain't Doin' Right"). And then the big question, "What do you think it is?" Of course the intent was to save the trouble of bringing the pet to the clinic and, more importantly, to save the cost of an exam. Some of those questions could be answered by my receptionist or tech, but most would require an examination in order to make an accurate diagnosis. In those cases, more often than not, the owner would make an appointment and then not show up.

Another challenge that I faced in the early days of practice was finding a way to eat at least two good meals a day when I was low on cash, which was most of the time. Finding good food was not the issue, but finding the cash to pay for it was. I wasn't steadily busy and when I did have work, I would usually send the owner a bill and it could take weeks or months before I would finally be paid. Fortunately there were three restaurants all within a mile or so of my clinic on Conley Road: Victor's Cafe at the Crossroads, The Farmer's Market also near the Crossroads, and The Riviera Restaurant about a mile up Doniphan from the Crossroads. All three opened early for breakfast and stayed open late for dinner.

Victor's had a great breakfast, the Farmer's Market had the best double meat bar-b-que brisket sandwich I have ever eaten, and the Riviera had the best Mexican food in town. Breakfast at Victor's, lunch at the Farmer's Market and dinner at the Riviera. And for a change, I would occasionally reverse the order. But, most importantly, each would let me charge. I'd sign an IOU after a meal and when I accumulated a little money I'd pay off as many of them as I could. This continued for quite some time. Their food was unbeatable and their prices were right. Without their help, aside from possibly starving, I probably would have given up on the idea of having my own practice and would have gone to work for another clinic for a guaranteed salary. Their help gave me more financial staying power to continue to work and build my practice.

Compared to today's fees, back in the '60's mine were awfully low. A dollar was worth more then than now, but the main reason that I survived was because of my low operating expense. I didn't need much income to pay my bills and have enough left over to cover my personal expenses. Here are some examples of my fees in early 1966 taken directly from my old day books:

    Small animal exam...$2
    Antibiotic injection...$2.
    Antibiotic/Steroid injection...$2.50
    Fecal exam (microscopic)...$1
    After hours caesarian section (dog)...$45
    Surgery to remove skin lesion small animal/local anesthetic...$5
    Farm call to treat horse for colic including tubing...$12.50
    Call to farm/pregnancy test 4 mares...$16
    Farm call and castrate horse...$25
    Tube deworm horse...$7.50
    Float teeth horse...$7.50
    Farm call/health certificate for horse...$7.50
    Farm call/treat cow with bloat...$12
    Rabies vaccination...$3
    DHL vaccination...$5
    Dog spay...$20
    Castrate cat...$7.50
    Cat spay...$15.00

Anyone who has purchased veterinary services recently will quickly recognize that today's fees are very different from those back in the day. My fees were lower than those of established practices simply because I needed the work and lower fees usually correlate with increased workload. I needed more transactions to keep busy and spread the word that I was new and available for work. From '66 through '68 I intentionally kept my fees lower than competing practices. Even though my fee structure changed little, my income grew by increasing my work load.

By 1968 my practice on Conley Road was growing and I was turning enough profit to live on (frugally) and then some. I was happy in El Paso and had no intention of leaving. I decided that it was time to build and own my clinic. I wanted a free-standing building in an area that offered good growth potential. Because of zoning issues with the city I had to move away from the Crossroads area. Coronado would have been a good location but city zoning issues also prevented that. I finally found a lot on Mesa Street between Coronado and Kern Place, just a few miles from Conley Road. That would be close enough to the Crossroads that I should be able to keep most of my small animal clientele from that area and also draw new clients from Coronado, Kern Place and Mission Hills. My large animal practice should not be affected since I did all of that work on a farm or ranch.

There were no residences in the immediate area of my proposed clinic at the time and the only business was a drive-in theatre directly across Mesa St. However, the zoning was appropriate for an animal clinic and I was certain that the area would eventually fill in with commercial and residential properties.

I contracted with Emilio Peinado, a developer/builder, for the small lot and a 1000 sf building to be built according to my plans. I signed a 5-year lease with Mr. Peinado and had an option to purchase. After one year of leasing, my practice was growing rapidly, so I exercised my option to purchase and thus began the next chapter of my career.

7

When All Else Fails

It was forecast to be well north of a 100 degrees in the summer of 1966, when I got a call from the owner of a small feedlot on the New Mexico side of the upper valley. He had a cow that was trying to deliver a calf, so far unsuccessfully, and wanted me to come out and take a look. I got there about noon and it was already plenty hot. Thankfully the air was dry, an element that makes the high, dry desert climate tolerable and, with a little shade and a light breeze, even comfortable in the heat of the day.

It was a small cattle feeding operation as far as feed lots go, with a capacity of a couple hundred head. It was also used as a holding facility for cattle coming out of Mexico enroute to larger feeders farther north and back in the midwest. It was located about a mile south of the Rio Grande River up in the sand hills where the nearest vegetation resembling a shade-producing tree was a mesquite bush. There were scattered yuccas, Spanish daggers and various types of cacti, not great shade-makers either.

Driving south on the dirt road after I turned off the pavement, Mt. Cristo Rey, with it's statue of Christ sitting on top, was no more than a mile or so off to my left and the mountains just west of Juarez were just a few miles south. It's a beautiful area in a rugged kind of way. The mountains and desert sand dunes were topographical features that attracted me to this country.

The feed lot was constructed of railroad cross-ties planted deep into the sandy soil and metal pipes that connected them. There was very little shade for what I estimated to be about 200 head of mixed, rangy-looking Mexican crossbred beef cattle. They were mostly steers, but there were also a few heifers. Mexican cattle were popular with U.S. feedlot operators because of their hardiness and ability to gain weight rapidly.

The sandy ground was already so hot I could feel the heat through the thin soles of my boots when I stood in one place for more than a few seconds.

The owner met me and directed me to a small holding pen where a cow was lying down on her side on the sand in the blazing sun. Her head was near a cross-tie in the middle of the pen and a wire stretcher was on the ground next to another cross tie about eight feet behind her. It took no genius to figure out that she was pregnant and had been in labor for who knows how long and was unable to deliver.

The presence of the wire stretcher made it pretty obvious that the owner and his cowboy helpers had been trying to "pull" the fetus from the cow's uterus, no doubt with the intention of saving the cost of a veterinarian. The cow's neck was tied to a cross-tie that was near her head in order to prevent her from being pulled across the sand by the stretcher that was attached to the legs of the calf on one end and anchored to a firmly-planted crosstie on the other. She was literally being pulled at both ends. She was perhaps unlucky to have survived the trauma that had been inflicted on her not to mention the dehydrating effect of the heat.

There was a water trough at the other end of the thirty foot long pen but it did her no good since she was unable to stand or walk. I saw no evidence that anyone had bothered to take a bucket of water to her either.

The owner and one of his cowboys told me that she had been in labor off and on for a couple days. After a day with no results they decided that maybe she needed more help. They applied the wire stretcher and after several unsuccessful attempts in which they said they exerted as much tension as they could, one of the fetus' legs was torn off its body. At that point they figured if it wasn't already dead, it would be shortly.

No problem though. They simply attached the stretcher to the other leg and soon ripped it off too. When the odor became so foul that they didn't want to mess with it anymore, they finally decided that maybe it was time to call the vet. When all else fails, call the vet.

The calf was dead and decomposing inside the uterus, and it probably had been dead for at least a couple days, perhaps longer. Most likely it died shortly after the cow began active labor which I was sure had to be two or three days ago, but the owner admitted to only one day of labor. The odor of the discharge from the birth canal made necropsy lab in vet school smell like a bouquet of roses.

My physical exam indicated that the cow was in amazingly good condition given all that she had been through for the last day or two. Her temperature was elevated, probably as much because of the direct sunshine and heat as the dystocia. She was unable to stand because a nerve that innervates her back legs had been traumatized to the point of paralysis by many attempts to deliver a fetus that was entirely too large to pass through the birth canal.

By now the owner and four of his cowboy hands were gathered around, offering no help at all, wanting only to see if the young vet had any idea what he was doing. I could tell they weren't very optimistic that I did. I was providing a little live entertainment for them before lunchtime. I sensed that they were hoping I could do no more than they had done and at the moment, I wasn't sure that I could. I usually enjoyed obstetrics but this was not going to be fun. I had to give it a try, though, for the cow's sake and because I needed to earn a fee. If I walked away from this stinking situation now, which surely would have been easy to do, the cow would have died a miserable death and I would have simply wasted half a day.

I catheterized a jugular vein and started a fast intravenous drip of a cool balanced electrolyte solution, put on a pair of coveralls and ob sleeves.

Working from a kneeling position on sand that must have been at least 110 degrees, I began to remove the fetus through the birth canal literally one small piece at a time. Every time I would get what felt like a good hold on part of its anatomy, it would tear off. Each of the back legs came out in at least two or three pieces. The skin pulled off the bones. The ears ripped off the head. It was one of the most repulsive procedures I have ever performed.

It took about an hour of hard labor to get all of the fetus out of the uterus. I was soaked with sweat and feeling a little lightheaded, probably from dehydration.

I sensed that the owner and helpers were probably disappointed that the live entertainment ended as soon as it did. It did not end too soon for me.

After removing the placenta and giving her an injection of oxytocin to help clean out her uterus, I loaded the poor cow up with antibiotic intravenously and inserted several antibiotic boluses into her uterus. At that point I wouldn't have given a nickel for her chance of surviving and I told the owner that. But after what she and I had just gone through, I wanted to give her the best chance possible. I instructed him to build a shade over her immediately and keep plenty of cool water and feed within her easy reach. I'll be back tomorrow to check on her, I told him as I walked back to my truck.

I returned daily for the next three days to give her intravenous antibiotic. By the second day, she was eating and drinking and walking around the pen. Her improvement and eventual recovery were nothing short of miraculous.

For all of that, I billed the owner for $35 which probably did not even cover my cost for the drugs I used and dispensed, not to mention my time. That fee was ridiculously low even for the 60's. I suspected that it was probably going to be difficult to collect my fee for this job. I was right. It took six months, several bills and a couple of threatening letters to finally collect.

Two good things resulted from this experience: the cow survived and it was a major learning experience for a young, naive vet who knew little, but was learning fast, about human misbehavior and the business of veterinary medicine. It also influenced my decision to eventually limit my practice to small animals, which I eventually did but not for a few more years, in spite of how much I enjoyed working with horses and cattle. I have often thought about and regretted not continuing large animal practice, especially horses. But it simply came down to the economics of veterinary practice. It's a profession, but it's also a business that must be managed wisely with an eye constantly on income and expense in order to have a chance to succeed.

I received a call one Saturday morning from a local oral surgeon who owned a ranch near

Dell City, Texas, which is about 100 miles east of El Paso. He had been notified that morning by his ranch manager that one of his most valuable bulls was down and the ranch hands were unable to get him up. They thought that he was going to die if he didn't get help fast. I agreed to take the case but it was Saturday morning and my clinic waiting room had clients who had been waiting for quite a while and I still had more appointments on my day book. In other words, I could not leave immediately and I advised the owner that I most likely wouldn't be able to leave till mid-afternoon. He asked if I would mind flying to his ranch and I told him that I wouldn't mind at all. Based on his description of the bull's signs I was pretty sure that I knew what medications I would need to take with me and I was sure that there would be enough room in the plane to carry everything.

I met the pilot, who also was my flight instructor for my private pilot license, at El Paso International Airport. He had the plane, a beautiful, almost new, Beechcraft Debonair that was being rented for this trip by the owner of the bull, all gassed up, pre-checked and ready to go as soon as I got there. That's a fast airplane and it didn't take us long to get there. We landed on a paved landing strip just outside of the small ranching community. One of the ranch hands was waiting for us and we loaded ourselves and my supplies and medications into his pickup. Upon arriving at the ranch there were three more cowboys sitting on a couple of bales of hay next to the bull. Each was chewing tobacco and picking his teeth with oat straw and wondering if this young whipper snapper vet had any idea what he was doing. I could tell that this was going to be another opportunity to provide some live entertainment.

The clinical signs and my physical exam pretty well confirmed my initial suspicion of what I would be dealing with here. After a couple liters of an intravenous fluid that I had brought and with a little encouragement, the bull got up and walked off and in short order started to graze. As they continued to spit tobacco and pick their teeth, the cowboys looked disappointed as their eyes shifted from the grazing bull, back to each other's face, then back to the bull, etc., etc. So much for their planned live entertainment.

8

Unconditional Love

It was mid-afternoon on a Sunday early in my career when my answering service called me at home with a message from a local doctor. This was before the founding of the Animal Emergency Clinic and very few vets took calls on Sunday, but I was still trying to build my practice so I took the call. He said his dog was bleeding and he thought that it was an emergency and asked if I would see her as soon as possible. It sounded like the dog needed help sooner than later so I agreed to meet him at the clinic in fifteen minutes. Callie was a nice little three year old, orange and white Brittany that I had seen a couple times for routine vaccinations. I remembered how easy she was to work with. She was always agreeable to whatever we needed to do. She never complained or resisted us.

The owner, who was wearing scrubs with the name of an El Paso hospital on the top, and his wife arrived shortly and carried Callie into the clinic. They both had blood on their clothes and the towel that she was wrapped in was soaked with blood. At first glance she appeared to be either heavily sedated or in shock or both. Her gums were pale, her heart rate was well above normal and her pulse was weak. She was covered with both clotted and fresh blood that was coming from what appeared to be an incision or perhaps a deep laceration on her mid-abdomen. It was a fresh wound with loose skin sutures that looked like they had been placed in a hurry. The hair had been clipped around the wound and I suspected that she had very recently had abdominal surgery and was now bleeding into her abdomen and the incision had opened enough to allow fresh blood in the abdomen to leak through. But the incision looked fresh, like maybe it was only a couple of hours old, and the sutures did not look like the kind of work a veterinarian would do.

My evaluation of this situation wasn't coming easy mainly because neither spouse was forthcoming with an explanation of what happened. They were both evasive and perhaps a bit fearful. The more I questioned them the more suspicious I became of foul play. Finally, I told them that she was in danger of dying soon and from what I could see it appeared that she was bleeding internally and would require sur-gery, as if they didn't already know that. I ex-plained that she would have a better chance to survive if I knew what had happened.

While I was waiting for one of them to open up and talk, I placed an intravenous catheter in a front leg vein and started dripping a balanced electrolyte solution and a fast-acting intrave-nous steroid for shock. Then I started oxygen flow via a mask that covered her muzzle.

The wife sheepishly and reluctantly finally began to talk. Callie had come into heat a few days ago and she had a blood-tinged dis-charge which normally occurs during that time. Her husband had gotten fed up with the blood around the house so instead of taking her to a vet clinic to fix the problem, which at this point I'm sure that he was wishing he had, he invited a doctor friend over to his house that morning to help him spay her, technically known as an ovariohysterectomy.

After the two discussed and planned the anesthesia and surgery, they were certain that this would be a piece of cake and fun too. Imagine how their colleagues would get a big kick out of this when they heard the story about how they spayed a dog in its owner's garage.

Now the doc began to talk. He was begin-ning to show signs of remorse and perhaps fear of losing his dog, not to mention the possibility for legal issues that might result if certain authorities, i.e., El Paso Animal Control, Texas State Board of Veterinary Medical Examiners and Texas State Board of Medical Examiners were to find out what he had done. He swallowed his pride and told me about the failed anesthetic and surgical procedure. For anesthesia he gave her an injection of a short-acting drug that in animals is mostly used for heavy sedation, but does not induce extended general anesthesia. It is suitable for certain brief, minor surgeries or procedures such as dental cleaning but not for longer, more painful surgeries such as ovariohysterectomy. After a short time she became sedate enough that they could tie her legs with her belly up on a work table in the garage. They used a general surgery pack that was provided by his doctor friend. At least he had sterilized it, which was about the only thing they had done correctly.

They had removed one ovary and were dissecting tissue from the horn of the uterus when Callie began to recover from the sedation, to the extent that they were unable to continue the surgery without another injection of the anesthetic. They had to physically restrain her for a few minutes while it took effect. While they waited for her to become sedated they noticed blood pooling in her abdomen, almost certainly indicating that a suture tie that they had applied to the blood supply to the ovary that they had removed had come off, or perhaps had not been adequately knotted and loosened. This can quickly lead to serious, often fatal hemorrhage.

This experience was suddenly not nearly as much fun as they had expected. They knew that they were in way over their heads and Callie needed help that they were not capable of giving. They were unable to find the bleeder inside the abdomen so they put the uterus and remaining ovary back into her belly and quickly closed the incision in her belly wall. That's when they called my answering service.

I was angry and did not try to hide it. The thought that these two highly trained medical professionals would even think of doing such a thing. Money for the surgery certainly was not the issue. And neither of them was working that particular day. At any rate, this was no time for a lecture. Callie needed help. I sent the two home and told them I would call as soon as I had something good or bad to tell them.

Then I called Edita for help. Fortunately, the bleeding seemed to be slowing, giving us a little more time to prep her for surgery. When she appeared to be somewhat stable we anesthetized her with an inhalant anesthetic/ oxygen mixture. The anesthesia and surgery were very risky because of shock, but I was certain that she had one or more major bleeders in her belly that were continuing to pump blood out of her general circulatory system. They had to be tied off or she would probably bleed to death.

The surgery went well. I suctioned free, pooling blood out of her abdominal cavity and quickly found the bleeder, tied it off and removed the other ovary and uterus. As soon as I finished closing the incision we turned off the anesthetic gas but continued the oxygen to help her wake up faster. We kept her on the surgery table for about a half hour so that we could continue to monitor her heart rate and oxygen blood level, both of which were improving quickly. We had a warm heating pad under her and another over her to prevent hypothermia. Within about an hour she was awake and her vital signs were stable. We put her in an oxygen cage and covered her with a heating pad. We continued the warm intravenous solution. A couple hours later she was awake, bright and alert and wagging her tail, almost always a good sign.

This couple did not deserve to get their dog back. I could have, should have and today would have reported this to local law authorities as animal abuse. Unfortunately when all of this occurred, laws and punishment for such misbehavior were not nearly as stringent and enforceable as they are today. But none of that would have helped Callie and I was pretty sure that this experience had been unpleasant enough that he would never again try anything so stupid. But there was one more thing that I could do to cement all of this securely into his memory.

I decided that the best way to make this experience memorable for him was to charge him a fee so high that he would never forget it and most certainly would not want those who he was so sure would get a good laugh about his ability as a dog surgeon to ever hear the real story, including the fee the vet charged him for saving his dog. When he picked her up two days later, I remember how happy she was to see him after he almost killed her. That surely must have been a classic example of what some would call "unconditional love". He most certainly did not deserve it. I was hanging out around the corner but in sight of the reception counter and it made my day to see the pained look on his face when he was presented with the bill. I thought he was going to go into shock. That was the best punishment that I could think of and it worked. I never saw him or his wife again, which suited me just fine.

9
Vail

There are quite a few occupational hazards in the veterinary profession that a practicing veterinarian must be willing to accept: dog and cat bites and scratches, being kicked by horses and cattle, physical contact with infectious feces, vomitus, urine, exposure to zoonotic diseases, just to name a few. If someone cannot accept with that reality, it might be best to consider another career.

This was an experience that I had involving one of the hazards that back in the day was not uncommon.

In the early 1970's the rabies outbreak in El Paso continued, although at a somewhat lower incidence than it was in the late 60's. I still had to be aware of the presence of the disease but I wasn't always as cautious as I should have been.

In early 1971, I was presented with a medium-sized, brownish mixed breed adult male dog which, according to the owner who lived on the western outskirts of El Paso near the New Mexico state line, was lethargic, drooling and had refused to eat or drink for a couple of days. To the owner's knowledge he had never been vaccinated. He freely roamed the desert that the home backed up to and had occasional contact with what the owner assumed were wild dogs. In fact, he had seen the dog with a small pack of wild dogs about two weeks previously.

His temperature was 105 degrees F, which is about 3 degrees above what we consider to be the upper limit of normal. He had difficulty walking, occasionally stumbling on his front legs, and was also weak in his back legs. Involuntary eye movement known as nystagmus was present in both eyes and his pupils failed to respond properly to light.

All clinical signs pointed to a neurologic condition. I immediately suspected a central nervous system viral disease, which with the history of no vaccinations would most likely be either distemper or rabies.

We were taught in vet school to always be cautious when examining the mouth or throat of an animal suspected of having rabies. Saliva from an infected animal is concentrated with the rabies virus, which is the reason that a bite by a sick animal is the primary mode of transmission to a susceptible animal or person. However, the virus can also be transmitted by inhalation and eye contact.

We were also taught that a foreign body such as a stick or bone that had become lodged in the mouth or throat could mimic rabies. To be certain that we don't confuse rabies with a foreign body, we must visually examine the mouth and throat and always wear gloves and face and eye protection when doing so.

I was hesitant to examine his oral cavity but I had to rule out a foreign body. I put on a pair of rubber exam gloves but simply forgot to put on a face mask and protective eyeglasses. I held the upper jaw with my left hand while pulling the lower jaw down with my right. My face was about 18 inches from the dog's mouth when it coughed twice directly into my face, splattering my eyes, nose and lips with thick saliva. I was able to get a good look into the oral cavity and did not see a foreign body. Then I quickly excused myself from the examination room and went directly to the restroom where I washed my face with soap and flushed my eyes with water and blew my nose for several minutes. There was no question that, if this animal was sick with rabies, I had just been exposed to the virus. My best hope was that it was not rabies but perhaps distemper, to which humans are not susceptible.

I finished my examination and advised the owners that there was a good possibility that the dog had rabies. Of course, that scared them and they did not want to return home with the dog, which I strongly advised against anyway. I recommended that we send the dog to animal control for quarantine and observation until it became more clear what was causing the sickness. They readily agreed and an animal control officer came that afternoon and picked up the dog.

A couple of days later Edita and I left for Vail, Colorado, where I had enrolled in a long weekend seminar in orthopedics. In addition to several hours of daily lectures by world-class veterinary orthopedists on the latest in orthopedic surgery, we also had the added pleasure of snow skiing for a couple hours daily. The seminar was Friday thru Sunday, but we planned to extend our stay by a couple more days.

I got a phone call on Saturday of the seminar weekend from one of my practice partners. Turns out the dog died the day after we sent it to animal control and the brain was sent to Austin for examination that same day. The results were phoned to animal control who in turn called the clinic: positive for rabies.

I contacted my personal doctor the same day and described to him exactly what had happened in the exam room. It had been several years since I had received a vaccination or even a titer check. He recommended that I get a blood draw for a rabies titer which would evaluate how strong my immunity was. That would require several days and in the meantime until we got the results of that test he wanted me to start anti-rabies treatment immediately. I guessed that I probably did have protective immunity but given my unquestionable exposure, I didn't want to take a chance on it.

I had to decide whether to leave Vail and the seminar and get back home as soon as I could or perhaps start the daily anti-rabies injections in Vail. I chose the latter option, assuming that I could actually start the injections there.

The Vail Clinic was established in the early 1960s as a general medicine/surgical clinic and by the time I arrived in the early '70's it was well on its way to becoming a world-renowned medical facility, especially in orthopedic surgery.

I arrived at the clinic the morning after I learned of the rabies positive diagnosis. I explained to the front office staff that I was a veterinarian and had been exposed to rabies. I needed to get a blood draw for a titer and start daily anti-rabies injections. I think that they first thought that I was joking with them. I finally convinced them that I was dead serious but they seemed to be somewhat bewildered with not much of an idea of where to start. In their defense, the Vail Clinic was world-renowned for its orthopedic surgery. Their clients were world-class athletes and celebrities who wanted the absolute best surgical care possible and the Vail Clinic delivered as I'm sure that it still does. They just did not appear to be prepared to deal with rabies.

After talking with a receptionist, two RN's and a physician, I finally convinced them that I wasn't kidding. They finally drew my blood and sent it by bus to Austin that same day. One goal accomplished, one to go.

I got the impression that this was the first time that the Clinic had been asked to administer the standard anti-rabies treatment which consisted of fourteen daily injections of rabies vaccine. Of course they had no rabies vaccine on hand and no idea where to get it. Finally, after calling a couple of their pharmaceutical/biological suppliers in Denver, they found the vaccine and ordered it to be sent by bus to arrive later that same day.

I was back at the Clinic late that afternoon to start my treatment. I had always wondered what the fourteen day treatment would be like, if it was really as painful as I had heard it was. I was about to find out. My first injection was subcutaneous on the left side of my abdomen. A little sting but not intolerable and the discomfort didn't last long. So far so good. Back the next day for another one, this one into my right abdomen. Same as the first, tolerable. By now the first injection site was red and painful to the touch. That night I had to sleep on my back or right side because of the pain in my left belly wall.

The next day the injection was given on the left side of my back. That night I couldn't sleep on my belly because of the pain of the first two injections. And so it went. Each injection had to be given in a different part of my body and after about 24 hours each injection site became quite painful to the touch. I realized that those who had told me that this was a painful treatment were not joking. The toughest part of the treatment was sleeping, or trying to sleep. It was difficult to find a position that I could sleep in that would not come in contact with the previous injection sites.

We were back home Wednesday of the following week and I continued the daily injections at my personal doctor's office. After nine injections I finally got the titer report which indicated that I had a protective level of immunity.

I stopped the daily shots at that point, which I was more than ready to do.

I was grateful to the Vail Clinic for starting my treatment and helping us stay there for a couple days of skiing after the seminar ended, but I must admit, I have never been more careful to avoid falling. The thought of falling and bouncing off one of the injection sites was more than enough to cause me to use great care in my ski technique.

An interesting side-note is the way Edita's grandfather, Dr. Hugh S. White, a pioneer El Paso physician who arrived in the early 1900's, treated rabies exposure in people. Rabies was rampant, not just in the immediate El Paso area but in northern Mexico as well. His reputation deep into Mexico was legendary and many people traveled from well south of the border for his care.

In those days El Paso was isolated and bio-logics companies and suppliers were few and far between. So, Dr. White produced his own rabies vaccine. He kept a stable of rabbits that he hyperimmunized by giving them frequent rabies vaccinations for an extended period. When he had given enough vaccine to induce a very high level of anti-rabies antibodies he would euthanize them, remove their brain and spinal cord and fix that tissue in a chemical mixture that, as I recall, contained formalde-hyde. After several days of soaking he would chop up the tissue into a very fine texture that could be administered through a fairly large needle. It was crude, but it worked and saved many lives.

And I thought the injections that I got were painful. I can only imagine how Dr. White's treatment must have felt. He also treated a lot of rattle snake bites, but that's another story.

10

Pink Panties

Golf balls, bones, sticks, coins, rocks, socks, fishing line and hooks, nails, tacks, needles and safety pins, etc, etc. Animals, especially dogs and cats, will swallow (or try to) just about anything that they can get in their mouth. It is almost miraculous how some animals are able to swallow a foreign body, manage to get it down the esophagus and into the stomach, and from there into the small intestine where it might or might not continue its movement down the gut into the colon and eventually be passed with a bowel movement. More often than not, however, a foreign body will lodge somewhere in the digestive tract and not move beyond that point. I never failed to be amazed by what I would see on radiographs of a chest or abdomen with a foreign body.

There are always exceptions but in most cases gastrointestinal foreign bodies do not cause serious illness as long as they either pass or are removed in a timely manner. One of the more common exceptions would be a foreign body that penetrates through the wall of the esophagus, stomach or intestinal tract and causes peritonitis. Those cases need immediate and aggressive treatment.

A typical foreign body case would be bright and alert, perhaps with non-specific vomiting or attempted regurgitation and perhaps a loss of appetite. But most cases would not appear to be downright sick. Diagnosis is fairly straightforward, often with the owners describing how they actually saw the animal swallow whatever it was that it should have left alone. And of course any diligent owner, seeing this happen, will make every attempt to get the animal to drop it out of their mouth and if that fails will open the animal's mouth and attempt to physically remove it. It's amazing how often all of this effort to prevent swallowing the foreign body almost guarantees that it's going to happen.

Treatment is also straightforward. If the foreign body is lodged in the upper gastrointestinal tract, i.e., the esophagus or stomach, depending on its size and shape, it can often be removed via endoscopy with no surgery required. Cases that are not suitable for endoscopy will usually require surgery. Unless it is a long-standing case with secondary illness such as peritonitis, most surgery cases are routine and uneventful and make a good recovery.

Dixie, a five year old spayed female Basset Hound, and her owner, an attractive woman probably in her mid-thirties, were at the clinic front door early in the morning waiting for us to open. From a distance Dixie looked perfectly healthy, bright, alert and responsive, but according to her owner she had been vomiting or attempting to regurgitate for the last couple days, usually shortly after a meal, and except for her slight loss of appetite she seemed to feel and act okay. She was current on her vaccinations and had always been in good health.

I didn't find much outside of normal limits on my physical exam, except that she was mildly dehydrated and slightly sensitive to my abdominal palpation, especially in the anterior abdomen. Her stomach felt slightly enlarged and had an unusual "mushy" feel which could have been residual food from her breakfast that morning. Her blood count and chemistry tests were normal. I recommended that we radiograph her belly to look for anything out of the ordinary and the owner agreed.

The only abnormal finding on the radiographs was a mildly increased density in the stomach. There were several possible diagnoses, but I was most suspicious of a foreign body.

We hospitalized her and started an intravenous drip of a balanced electrolyte solution in order to rehydrate her. We then gave her a swallow of barium to help us firm up our tentative diagnosis.

The following morning we repeated the radiographs. Most of the barium had moved down the intestine into the colon but a considerable amount remained in the stomach. This supported my suspicion that there was a mass of some sort in the lumen of the stomach. I still felt that a foreign body was the most likely. Because of my uncertainty of the diagnosis, I recommended an exploratory laparotomy rather than gastroscopy to confirm my diagnosis and hopefully find a curable condition. The owner agreed.

We did not give Dixie breakfast that morning in anticipation that we might do surgery later that day. I decided that sooner was better later for the exploratory surgery, so we decided to get it done during our regular lunch time that same day. For general anesthesia we used propoflo, an ultra short-acting intravenous agent that is commonly used in human anesthesia, to induce anesthesia just deep enough to intubate her with a tracheal tube. We then hooked her up to our inhalation anesthetic machine in which we were using isofluorane, a safe anesthetic with rapid induction and recovery characteristics. We monitored her heart rate and blood oxygen level with a pulse/oximeter, also commonly used in human surgery.

We entered her belly with a four inch incision which allowed for good visualization of her entire abdominal cavity. The only abnormal finding was sure enough a palpably soft mass that occupied about one-third of her stomach capacity. A four inch incision into the stomach wall revealed foreign material that appeared to be cloth-like, perhaps silk. I removed it intact with no adherence to the inner stomach wall, which appeared to be somewhat inflamed but essentially normal. I handed the material to my tech and she took it out of the room to clean it and hopefully identify it. In the meantime I started my closure of the incisions into the stomach and abdominal wall. Just as I finished my closure and began to wake up Dixie, my tech returned holding up the clean foreign object so that I could clearly see that it was a pair of women's panties, at one time probably pink and still somewhat so except faded due to the effect of the stomach acid.

I called the owner after Dixie was awake and stable and told her that all was well and that she needed to come in to the clinic so that we could show her what we found. When she arrived about thirty minutes later, the tech took her into an exam room and showed her the pink panties, which were about the same color that her face had suddenly become. She was embarrassed but happy that Dixie was doing well. She called us shortly after she returned home and told us that, yes, she was missing a pair of pink panties, no doubt the pair that Dixie had consumed.

Dixie's appetite was beginning to return the following morning, so we started her on a bland, highly digestible diet. She recovered well and we sent her home the following day.

11

Fainting

In the early 1970's the rabies outbreak in El Paso continued but at lower incidence that it was in the 60's. Veterinarians still had to be cautiously aware of the presence of the disease.

I was presented with a medium sized, brownish, mixed breed male dog which, according to the owners, was lethargic, had no appetite and had been drooling for no obvious reason for a couple of days. They could not remember his ever having been vaccinated and he frequently left his yard and roamed through the neighborhood and adjacent desert.

His temperature was 105 F, which was about 3 degrees above the upper limit of normal, and occasionally stumbled on his front legs and weak in his hindquarters. The clinical signs suggested a neurological condition, probably a viral encephalitis. With his history and the incidence of the disease in the area at the time, I had to put rabies at the top of the list of differential diagnoses. Using a pair of exam gloves I got a good look in his mouth and throat and quickly ruled out foreign body.

Back in the exam room I explained to the anxious owners, who by now knew what I was thinking even though I had not yet told them, that rabies topped the list of possible causes of their pet's sickness. As soon as the word "rabies" left my mouth, the child who accompanied them and who I guessed was about ten years old, fainted and dropped to the floor. A good-sized lump appeared almost immediately on his forehead where it had bounced off the tile floor. I was praying that it was not a fractured skull.

After what seemed like a half hour of unconsciousness, but in fact was probably only a few seconds, he began to recover and even though he was dazed he was able to sit up. I recommended that we call an ambulance but his family declined, promising that they would go straight to a doctor from my office.

To err on the side of caution, I sent the dog to animal control with instructions to send the brain to Austin for rabies exam. The results came back in a couple of days: negative for rabies. I then suspected that distemper was the most likely cause of the clinical signs. I kept in touch with the owners for a few days and the child recovered completely.

The morning after that experience, I called my insurance carrier and substantially increased my liability insurance coverage.

A similar incident occurred in my office within a couple of months of the child's injury. Only this time it involved a Texas Western College (now the University of Texas El Paso) football player who accompanied his girlfriend and her sick dog. The guy was a giant. He was an offensive lineman and he must have weighed 250-300 pounds and stood at least 6'4".

I wasn't able to diagnose the dog's illness with a physical exam, so I recommended a blood test. The girl held the dog while I applied a tourniquet to his front leg. He had a good vein which I had no trouble hitting with a 20 gauge needle. I had about 4 ml of blood pulled into the syringe when I noticed the guy swaying back and forth, holding onto the exam table trying to keep from falling. His face was white as a ghost, drained of blood. I knew he was about to go but before I could tell him to sit down and lower his head, he hit the deck almost pulling the exam table over on top of himself. He was out like a light.

The girl became frantic and started to scream. Now I have a sick dog pouring blood from the venipuncture site, an out of control young lady and out cold college offensive lineman to deal with. At this point the canine was in better shape than the two homo sapiens, so I loosened the tourniquet and quickly put a piece of cotton over the blood gusher and firmly told the young lady to stop screaming and press on the cotton while I attended to her friend. I had recently purchased a bottle of smelling salts for exactly such an occasion. Within seconds I had it under his nose and within a few more seconds he was turning his head away from it. I didn't see any physical evidence of injury, but I knew this guy was going to have to get up on his own, since he weighed 150 pounds more than I did.

Within a minute or so he was able to sit up but I insisted that he stay on the floor with his head down between his legs for a while.

I rubbed his face and the back of his neck with a cold, damp towel for a couple minutes while the color slowly returned to his face. Finally, he was able to stand up and appeared to be completely back to normal, albeit embarrassed.

Now back to the canine patient. By now the blood in the syringe had clotted so I needed to do another venipuncture. The young lady was apologetic but okay and again agreed to hold the dog while I drew blood. Before I pulled out another syringe and needle, I suggested to the offensive lineman that it might be best if

he left the room this time. He quickly accomo-
dated, vacating not only the room but the entire building.

Another incident involving fainting occurred
when a woman and her son, who I guessed was
nine or ten years old, came in to the clinic with
a sick dog. It was a one year old mixed breed
female, no appetite for a couple days and was
coughing. No change in its behavior other than
lethargy and a low grade fever. It had a purulent
discharge from its eyes and nose. The owner
showed me documents that confirmed that the
dog had been vaccinated appropriately for rabies but never finished the initial series of distemper vaccinations.

Several cases of rabies had been recently
reported and the word was spreading fast that
if you had a sick dog, regardless of the clinical signs and vaccination history, by all means
get it to a vet asap. I could tell that the mother
and boy were quite concerned about their pet's
sickness, especially the possibility of rabies.
She was standing at the exam table holding the
dog and her son was a few feet away standing
quietly with his hands folded behind his back.
He hadn't said a word.

I did not find anything on my physical exam
that made me suspect rabies but, because I
always felt the need to cover my back side,

with all the rabies we were seeing in the area at the time, I would never completely exclude it from the list of differential diagnoses. I felt that I needed to say or do something that would relieve her anxiety a bit. I ran down the list of possible causes of her pet's sickness and finished by saying that although I didn't strongly suspect rabies, it too would be on the list of possibilities. As soon as I said "rabies" the boy immediately fainted and dropped in his tracks.

After a few whiffs of smelling salts, he came around and could sit up. I encouraged him to sit for a while and after about ten minutes helped him to his feet. He was able to stand and walk with no obvious lingering effects. I suggested to the mother that if she was concerned about him in any way that she should not hesitate to take him to their family doctor.

After thinking about it for a day or two, I suspected that the family had been discussing the possible causes of their pet's sickness and no doubt rabies had been mentioned. The boy was old enough to understand the seriousness of the disease and how it could be fatal not just in the animal, but to people as well. No doubt he loved the dog and was much more appre-hensive than I realized at the time. He was also concerned about his own health and my simply saying the word "rabies" was all it took for him to faint.

I treated the dog for an upper respiratory infection, possibly a mild case of distemper, and it recovered uneventfully.

Fainting under such circumstances is usually embarrassing, especially if the victim happens to be a veterinarian with eight years of practice experience under his belt. That's right, it happened to me while I was in graduate school at Colorado State University. My timing could not have been worse.

It happened while I was assisting Henry Swan, MD, perform an aortic stenosis repair in a dog. Dr. Swan was a world-renowned chest surgeon on the faculty of the University of Colorado medical school. He was also a faculty member at CSU where he taught graduate level veterinary thoracic surgery and conducted research. He was the innovator of open chest cardiac massage as a treatment for cardiac arrest. He was a genius, not only as a surgeon but as a thinker. The opportunity to work shoulder to shoulder with him in surgery was an honor.

We were about an hour into the surgery when I became light-headed and started seeing brightly-colored stars shooting across my field of vision. Then I began to sweat profusely, soaking my cap, mask and gown. My big chance to work with Dr. Swan and I was about to blow it. As discreetly as I could, given the situation, I began to quietly hyperventilate and I lowered my head to below my shoulder level. That was all I could do short of sitting down on the floor at the surgery table. It didn't help. I fought it as long as I could but I knew if I continued standing, I would pass out and drop to the floor. You can bet I'd never assist him again.

My only choice was to leave the table and worry about the consequences later. Fortunately, there was another assistant surgeon at the table who could pick up the slack. I left the table without saying anything. Dr. Swan was explaining what he was doing to the ten or so observers, my classmates, who were standing around the table. I went straight to the dressing room and lay down on a bench as soon as I got inside the door. After a couple of minutes I began to feel better. I washed my face and changed into dry scrub clothes. I quickly put on a new cap and mask, rescrubbed, regowned and as inconspicuously, and sheepishly as possible walked back into the surgery suite fully expecting to be told to leave.

I was absent from the table maybe ten to fifteen minutes total, and when I returned Dr. Swan was still explaining the hemodynamics, anesthesia considerations and other technical aspects of the hypothermia procedure. He never looked up as I resumed my work at the table. He was so completely preoccupied with what he was doing that I don't think he was aware that I had left and then returned. If he was, he fooled me. He never mentioned it. I did have to do some pretty heavy explaining later to the other assistant and the observers. I told them I thought I was coming down with the flu, or whatever. Anything but fainting.

That experience actually put me in pretty good company. A young lady friend of our family who had recently finished her bachelors in college came to the clinic one morning to observe surgery. She was experienced with horses and considering applying for veterinary school. I don't remember the procedure that I was doing but about halfway through it she became light-headed and began to get pale in the face. I asked her to leave the room and sit down for a few minutes. She recovered quickly and came back into the room and apologized and watched me finish with no further problem.

This apparently had no lasting negative effect on her. She went on to graduate from vet school with honors, got a PhD in her specialty and ultimately became a full professor and equine specialist at one of the top vet schools in the country.

12

Family

There is no question that people can become so close to animals that they consider them to be part of the family. It is commonly said that a pet is a "member" of the family, usually referring to a dog or cat and occasionally to a back yard type horse. I've seen many animals over the years that absolutely were an integral part of the family structure. Seldom, however, is it said that a milk cow is a member of the family, but it happens.

While still working for Dr. Butchofsky at The Animal Clinic, I was making my large animal rounds one day when I was sent to look at a sick cow near Fabens, a small town in El Paso's lower valley. When I arrived I was met by Mr. Dominguez, the owner of the cow and father of the two young children with him. They met me in the driveway of their small adobe home which sat on what I guessed was about an acre of land.

The four of us walked to the small barbed-wire pen behind the house where the cow, whose name was Billie, and a weaned calf were kept. I didn't see any other animals on the property. While Mr. Dominguez gave me as much history as he could, the two kids were hugging, patting, rubbing on and talking to her. One of the kids offered her a handful of grain and the other offered a small bunch of hay, both of which she refused. The dad explained, in an almost apologetic manner, that the family was quite worried about her and that she was a "member of the family" but, as happens all too often, they were limited in how much they could spend on her.

She had not been doing well for several days. Her appetite was off and she was listless, hardly moving at all unless she was made to do so. She had also lost quite a bit of weight recently and was having trouble breathing. They at least wanted a vet to look at her and hopefully help her. Besides being a friend to the family, she also provided milk for them. There was not only an emotional attachment, but she also helped to feed the family.

A quick look even from a distance and I could tell that she didn't feel good and appeared to be depressed. Her head and neck were extended and she was taking short, choppy breaths. Her jugular vein was distended and she had edema (subcutaneous fluid) under her neck and brisket. I listened to her chest with my stethoscope and found her heart sounds to be somewhat muffled with an elevated heart rate. She also had a fever.

I noticed right away that there were pieces of barbed and baling wire and broken glass scattered around the pen. They put her daily ration of grain in a barrel cut down to about a third its normal height and twice daily gave her a block of hay on the ground.

I had seen two cases of traumatic pericarditis, commonly known as "hardware disease", in cattle during my last two months of vet school and that experience proved to be helpful. The condition is caused by ingesting a piece of wire or nail or other metal object that gets mixed up with the grain or hay and is then eaten along with the feed. The metal then punctures through the intestinal tract and penetrates into the pericardium, the membrane that surrounds the heart. It causes infection and fluid accumulation inside the pericardial sac and compresses the heart, thereby compromising its function.

I was certain of my diagnosis and explained to Mr. Dominguez that the prognosis for her recovering from hardware disease was poor. He was saddened and concerned how he would explain this to his wife and children. I felt sorry for the family knowing how important Billie was to them. I offered to leave a couple of antibiotic-filled syringes at no cost to him, but I also told him that I did not expect her to improve. He accepted the syringes and I showed him how to administer it. I told him to call the clinic if he had questions. We never heard from him again.

Whether or not one approves or even agrees with me, I'm certain that in many families a pet is every bit as important as any of its blooded members. Based on my experience, it seems to me that considering and treating a pet as a real member of the family is much more common today than it was over fifty years ago. That's not to say that they weren't loved and cared for back in the day, there's just a stronger emotional attachment to pets in today's society.

I had a client with a small mixed breed female dog that had a chronic problem with contact dermatitis and its many clinical signs, such as intense itching and recurring skin infections. It was much worse during the warmer months but never went away completely even during the fall and winter. One of the most common causes of this condition in the El Paso southwest is bermuda grass and sure enough that was the grass that the pet owners had in their front and back yards where she spent a lot of time. The best long-term treatment for contact dermatitis is to remove the cause from the pet's environment, and I suggested to the owner that preventing her from coming in contact with bermuda grass would help alleviate, if not completely eliminate, her skin condition. The owners did not commit to such a radical and costly treatment, which was clearly understandable, so I sent them home with a medicated soap and an antihistamine.

I saw the little dog back about three to four months later and to my amazement her skin condition had almost completely cleared up. I knew that the medicated shampoos and antihistamines would help but I didn't expect to see that much improvement. The owner had hired a lawn service to remove every bit of the bermuda grass in both front and back yards. They replaced it with an ornamental rock. And there she was, almost like new. She was a much happier dog and the owner was also happy, in spite of the several thousands of dollars they spent. Not everyone can or will go to the trouble and expense that this owner did, but amazingly many will. Never underestimate the strength of the emotional attachment between man and animal.

El Paso is fortunate to have several animal rescue organizations, the Humane Society of El

Paso and El Paso Animal Services, and I'm fortunate that I got to work with many of them at one time or another, beginning in the 1960's for the city and the humane society. Many of the dogs and cats that I cared for were adopted from one of these organizations and turned out to be the best patients that I ever had. It was difficult to understand why an owner would relinquish their ownership only to have them adopted out. There were many reasons but I believe the most common was the owner's inability to adequately provide for the pet due to financial hardships.

I've often wondered who got the better side of an adoption, the adoptee or the adoptor. Each seemed to appreciate the new relationship. Reminds me of a bumper sticker that I saw a while back. It reads: "Who Rescued Who?" A "rescue" can and often does work both ways.

Then there's the opposite extreme of responsible pet ownership. I did some work for a pet shop/groomer who kept a fairly small inventory of dogs and cats in his shop for retail sale. He did his own vaccinating for everything except rabies, which was required by law to be given by a veterinarian. So my work with him was limited to an occasional rabies vaccination or sickness, usually the type that is most likely to occur in overcrowded, unsanitary conditions.

He was slow to pay and I threatened many times to stop working for him.

One day he came to the clinic with six mixed breed puppies, about two months old. They all appeared to be in good health. I asked him why he was there. Well, he said, after a couple weeks of trying he had been unable to sell them, was tired of feeding and taking care of them and, therefore, losing money on them. He wanted me to euthanize them. I had to leave the room before I blew my top and said something that might have resulted my having to defend myself before the State Board.

I gathered my emotions and walked back into the exam room. I told him that he couldn't pay me enough to euthanize those puppies. He could take them to city Animal Control or Humane Society where they would probably be adopted out. I made it clear to him that I didn't need his business and if I never saw him again it would be fine with me. I don't remember ever seeing him again.

Another example of someone who did not deserve to have a pet was a local physician who had been into the clinic a couple times for vaccinations. I didn't like him from the first time I saw him. He was cavalier and had what some would call a "god complex". He called the clinic one day and announced that his dog had gotten out of her yard and had anyone reported seeing her or perhaps brought her in as a stray. The answer was "no" but Edita immediately went to work making frequent phone calls to all of the rescue leagues and Animal Control Center doing what she could to help find the lost dog.

This went on for a couple of weeks and about when we were ready to give up we got a call from animal control that she had been found and delivered to them and that she had been identified by her microchip. She immediately got on the phone to the owner and left a message at his office that she had been found. He called back later that day and when told the good news about his dog his response was "I never liked her much anyway. Tell them to keep her and do whatever they want with her. Besides, I could buy another one for less than I would have to pay animal control to bail her out".

Euthanasia is an extremely stressful and emotional issue that veterinarians must deal with.

I'm sure that most practitioners would agree that it's not an easy topic to discuss, much less to perform. Euthanasia ends the life of, in most cases, a valued member of the family. It should never be viewed as just another fee transaction.

Even if it is a merciful procedure that brings untreatable, lingering pain and sickness to an immediate end, it is one of the most stressful aspects of practice that I had to deal with. It's difficult for some, perhaps not so much for others. I'm in the former group.

I am not a warm and fuzzy, touchy, feely, outgoing kind of person. Perhaps those who are are better suited to deal with the emotions of the moment. I never knew what to say to the client at such a difficult time for them. I tried to stay "at arm's length", isolated and unaffected by the emotions of the moment. The best I could do was say something to hopefully help the client know that he or she made the right decision in choosing euthanasia and had given the pet a wonderful life and to tell them that I respected and admired them for being such caring owners. Seldom did I find the right words when I needed them.

I finally decided that what worked best for me was to simply say "I'm sorry" and then leave the room to give the remaining family members time to say "goodbye".

Veterinary practice is physical work. Staying in good physical condition helps to maintain a heavy workload and it helps to prevent injuries to the practitioner, which, unfortunately, are to be expected, especially in large animal work.

I was on a call to an upper valley farm to tube deworm several head of horses. Tubing a horse typically is not difficult, especially if you are dealing with a cooperative animal. It's not a completely safe procedure, though, given that you are standing directly in front of the horse's head and front legs which some horses are pretty handy with. There is always a certain degree of vulnerability, especially if the horse rears up and thrashes out at you with its front hooves, sometimes making physical contact. The procedure usually does not require sedation, but I would almost always put a twitch on the horse's upper lip and then have the twitch holder twist it just enough to distract the animal. I used a clear plastic, lubricated tube that was long enough to go through the nose, into the esophagus and all the way down to the stomach. After entering the esophagus I could usually actually see the end of the tube as I gently pushed it farther down into the stomach.

When I was sure that I had the tube in the stomach, I attached a small hand pump to the other end of the tube and pumped the deworming solution directly into the stomach. The entire process would take only a few minutes.

I was on a farm call in the upper valley one day to tube deworm several head of horses. I had completed a routine deworming via stomach tube in a nice quarter horse that the owner's daughter rode competitively in barrel racing. As I was removing the tube from her stomach, with no warning whatsoever, the mare jumped straight up on her back legs and came toward me thrashing out with her front hooves. I could not get out of her way fast enough to avoid contact. She hit me with the toe portion of a hoof about an inch under my lower lip. Then she immediately settled as if nothing had happened. I pulled the rest of the tube out and we removed the twitch. She was fine, but I wasn't.

I had about an inch and a half long laceration that paralleled my lower lip between it and the point of my chin. I went to my truck and checked it in a mirror. Except for being dirty and bloody, it was a clean cut which I could stick the tip of my tongue through. I applied pressure and finally got the bleeding stopped and finished deworming the rest of the horses. The owner felt bad about it and offered to pay for medical treatment. I thanked him but it wasn't his fault. That sort of thing happens. I went straight to my doctor's office, which at the time was at the Johnstone Clinic in Ysleta, on the southeast fringe of El Paso. After numbing me up the nursing staff cleaned it and my doctor (Ed Jabalie, MD) did a skillful job of suturing it, both inside and outside my mouth. After a tetanus vaccination and a prescription for antibiotic and pain medication, I was on my way back to my clinic where I had several small animal clients waiting.

A similar incident occurred while I was tube deworming one of my own horses. Zorro was his name and I used him for polo which he didn't care for. Nor did he like me. I wasn't particularly fond of him either. I had a helper apply a twitch on his upper lip and about the time that I had the tube about halfway down his esophagus en-route to his stomach when he reared up and came down thrashing out at me with both front legs. This time a front hoof hit me with a downward glancing blow that left a deep abrasion on the tip of my nose. If I had been about a half inch closer to him, it would have broken my nose, or worse.

Dorado was a palomino who stood about fifteen hands and had the appearance one would expect of a quarter horse, although coming from Mexico we couldn't be sure. He was given to my father-in-law, Wyndham K. White, by a friend of his, Tom Beall, who lived in El Paso but had a ranch in Mexico. Dorado was brought up from Chihuahua along with a two-year-old quarter horse filly named Tomasa, one of the sweetest horses I ever met. Tomasa had a running W brand on her hip, which of course is the King Ranch brand, and we never figured out why or when she got it. Dorado had a horseshoe brand (heels pointed down) on one hip. On the other hip was a 2 which signified that he had been foaled in 1952. We assumed that both Dorado's brands were those of a Mexican ranch but we never knew for sure.

Dorado had been at the Mexican cavalry detachment in Delicias, Chihuahua, Mexico. Many good riders came from there to El Paso to compete in the shows that were held at the El Paso County Coliseum during the 1960's.

Dorado and Tomasa were shipped to Juarez and crossed the border. Mr. White went to pick them up at the stockyards in El Paso and Dorado refused to load into the trailer. Someone came up behind him and whacked him hard with a 2 X 4 sending him into the trailer on top of Mr. White, who had no quick, easy way out. He curled up in a ball to protect himself as the horse scrambled around inside the trailer. Mr. White was finally able to get out of the trailer but he always remembered seeing the hooves clattering around his head as he crawled out.

When they finally unloaded at the White's house, Dorado wanted nothing to do with anyone. When he was turned loose, he went to the farthest side of the corral and put his head in the corner and would not even turn around to look at anyone.

The day that Mr. White rode him for the first time he had an attorney colleague and friend in attendance to watch the action. The friend, who was also a horseman, became so nervous about the first ride on a difficult and probably dangerous horse that he went behind the barn and threw up. Mr. White was able to carefully and quietly get on Dorado and miraculously he didn't buck at all. He concluded that the horse had been well-trained and ridden but had been badly abused on the ground and trusted no one, especially adults. The only way they could catch him was to gently ease him up to a fence and softly ease a lead rope over his neck. When he felt the rope on his neck he would stand still and accept a halter without resistance.

As Hugh, my brother-in-law, put it "if you were quiet and fair with him you could talk him into anything. But if you tried to get after him he would fight back."

After Mr. White had ridden him enough to get to know him, the kids in the family took over. Anne, Hugh and Breezy, Edita's three siblings, all competed on him in several shows here and in Arizona and did quite well. The horse trusted and liked kids.

Eventually word got back to the Whites that

Dorado had been sent or possibly sold to the army unit in Delicias and while at the post one of the soldiers had gotten into an altercation with him in a stall. Speculation was that perhaps the soldier was "teaching him a lesson". What he didn't know was that the horse was very fast and aggressive with his front feet. He got the man down in the stall and killed him. The commanding officer had Dorado shipped out to El Paso that day out of fear that if he stayed overnight the other soldiers would kill him to avenge their friend.

Hugh was grooming him while at a show at the coliseum. Dorado was tied to the trailer and a couple of the soldiers from Chihuahua walked by, stopped and looked at him very carefully and one of them said, "Matahombre", espanol for Mankiller.

As difficult and dangerous as he could be, he was loved by the Whites and helped to teach lots of little kids how to ride.

What does all this have to do with veterinary medicine? It's a classic example of the kind of behavior that a practicing vet must deal with at times. Dr. John Neal, one of the most competent equine specialists in El Paso, or anywhere else for that matter, attempted to treat Dorado once and was having a tough time with him when he was heard to say "I've cussed you and

I've wished you were dead, but I can't let the screwworms eat you!" And possibly the most difficult and potentially dangerous treatment that I can remember doing on a horse was when I was able to get a stomach tube down him once when he had colic. Fortunately he got well with only one treatment but from that time on every time he saw me, regardless how far away I was from him, he'd go to the far end of the corral and turn his back side to me.

(Thanks to Hugh White, horse trainer and riding instructor in northern California for providing the information about Dorado.)

I was floating the teeth on a horse that I had twitched with my assistant, who was excellent with large animals, on the twitch. I was not using a speculum, which is a piece of equipment we use to keep the mouth open for a dental procedure or oral surgery. I would shortly come to regret that decision. I had my left hand about wrist deep into the right side of his mouth between his teeth and cheek and was palpating the sharp edges on the jaw teeth and talking to the horse owner at the same time. I was distracted and not paying attention when my left index finger got caught in between the upper and lower jaw teeth on the right side of the mouth. And then he closed his jaws. I could not remove my finger until I yelled and jumped at him. That scared him just enough to open his jaws which allowed me to remove my finger. My first thought was that the bone was crushed from about the third joint to the tip of the bone.

Another trip to my doctor where an x-ray showed that the bone was not crushed. That made me feel a little better but the concern now was that the blood supply to the tip of my finger had been compromised to the point that I might lose the tip anyway. After a local anesthetic, the wound was cleaned and the doctor placed several sutures to reattach the tip. The biggest challenge was trying to work, especially surgery, for the next couple of weeks with a splint on my left hand. After a few days the color of the skin over the tip of my finger had become nice and pink and there was no indication of infection. The wound healed well and I learned a lesson that stayed with me for the rest of my career: PAY ATTENTION and ALWAYS use a speculum when floating teeth on a horse.

It is an unusual dog or cat that is not stressed out when in a clinic environment. They go into a defensive mode to protect themselves and that is when bites and scratches are most likely to occur.

I was bitten by a dog once that almost tore my thumb nail off. Once again I had to deal with the challenge of working, especially surgery, with a thick bandage on my hand. But that's nothing compared to what happened to one of my techs. We had a nine month old Rottweiler on the treatment table for an examination. We had seen her several times only for routine matters, such as vaccinations, starting at about two months of age. She had always been friendly and we had never had any behavioral issues with her. One of my techs was holding her head and consoling her while I did a routine physical exam.

For some reason she turned her head abruptly in a way that caused the tech to lose her grip on her head. She bit at the tech's face and literally lacerated one side of her nose from her face. It all happened so quickly that the tech did not have time to move to safety. I sent the tech immediately to an urgent care center, where she got the wound repaired with many stitches. She healed fine and we never saw the dog back.

Then there was the little Peke that would begin to bite and chew on her owner's arm as soon as she was picked up to enter the clinic front door, not only leaving teeth marks but drawing blood. To the lady's credit she would not put her down on the floor but continue to hold and talk to her and try to comfort her while her arm was being mauled.

Another bite incident occurred but this time involved my oldest child, who at the time was about five years old. He had been spending time with me at my clinic. A dog that I had just vaccinated was on the floor walking around the exam room when Lito reached out to pat it. The dog bit him on a finger and caused enough of a laceration that we ended up shortly at an urgent care center for stitches.

In veterinary medicine, injuries do occur. Most minor, some serious. As unfortunate as they are, they are greatly outweighed by all the good things that also occur.

13

Orthopedics

Fracture cases, especially in small animals, were common in the late 1960s and early 1970s, partly because many pet owners ignored existing leash laws that were not being rigidly enforced. As a result, an increasing number of dogs and cats were brought to the clinic with injuries caused by HBC (hit by car). Many were soft tissue injuries only, such as abdominal and chest, but most also had an orthopedic component, such as a fracture or joint dislocation. Some of the simpler fractures were treatable with external fixation, such as splints and casts. More complicated cases required internal fixation, such as intramedullary pinning, which was probably the most widely-used form of internal fixation at the time.

I got a lot of experience with most forms of repair techniques and came to rely more and more on intramedullary pinning, an internal fixation technique in which one or more stainless steel pins are placed into the medullary canal of the broken bone after normal realignment is established. It worked well in most cases and the necessary equipment and implants were reasonably priced so that most owners could afford it. But IM pinning still left a lot to be desired especially in fractures involving several major bone fragments and smaller chips. I enjoyed the challenge of small animal orthopedics, fracture repair in particular, and wanted to learn more about some of the newer internal fixation techniques. I attended seminars that were heavy in orthopedics, including one in San Francisco, a couple in Vail, Colorado, and several in Texas.

I would go out of my way to attend a seminar in which Don Piermattei, DVM, PhD, was a speaker. I got to know him while I was in vet school at A&M. He was, as I recall, working on his Masters degree in surgery at the time and had a teaching position. He taught surgery to my class and ultimately he became one of the world's renowned veterinary surgeons.

Dr. Piermattei was not just smart, he was brilliant. I worked with some excellent surgeons, DVM and MD, during my career but I have never seen anyone better than him. I followed his work and purchased his books. He inspired me to continue learning as much as

I could about orthopedic surgery. I considered him a mentor, as did many aspiring surgeons back in the day.

In the early 1970s I attended the annual course on Internal Fixation of Fractures, including the theoretical basis and the practical application of bone healing and fracture repair, presented by the College of Veterinary Medicine at The Ohio State University, Columbus, Ohio. It was a three day course and was packed with information that I had not yet been exposed to. The Faculty included DVM and MD surgeons and again, as I recall, Dr. Piermattei was one of the presenters.

The OSU course concentrated on a relatively new, at least for the veterinary profession, methodology for internal fixation. It was developed for use in people by the Association for the Study of Internal Fixation, commonly known as the ASIF, and involved the use of metal implants, i.e., screws, plates and other implantable devices which could be removed after healing was complete or, in some cases, could be left in permanently. It wasn't long before its applications in veterinary surgery became obvious.

This new method of fracture repair was exciting. There was, however, going to be a downside to its use. It was much more expensive than Steinman pins, Kirschner wire and external fixation apparatus, Jonas pins, etc., and all the various types of splints that been the mainstays for fracture repair in animals. The upside was that it would eliminate several issues that we had with those methods.

Upon returning home from the OSU course, I ordered a basic ASIF kit which I received within few days. Shortly, I had my first case which, on radiograph, looked to be a perfect fit for my first surgery using the ASIF technique. It was a one year old female, mixed breed dog, weighing about twenty pounds. She had been hit by a car about an hour before coming to the clinic. The radiograph revealed a simple, mid-shaft, transverse fracture of the left radius (foreleg). She had a few bruises and abrasions but no other serious injuries.

We immobilized her leg with a Robert Jones splint which is a thick cotton bandage that is quite comfortable and easy to apply. We use it to minimize movement at the fracture site and lessen pain. Animals tolerate it very well. Her pre-anesthetic blood workup was perfect, so we hospitalized her and scheduled the surgery for the next morning.

Long story short, the surgery could not have gone better. I applied a plate to the bone, centered it over the fracture site and secured it with three screws above and three screws below the fracture site. I was able to get some compression at the fracture site, which allows for some weight-bearing on the fractured leg which, in turn, enhances healing. The post-op radiograph showed near perfect alignment. We applied another Robert Jones splint by the time we got her back in the cage she was beginning to wake up.

The owner came the next morning to pick her up and I let her walk out of the kennel room up to the reception area to greet her owner. She was well-behaved and I felt certain that weight-bearing on the leg would enhance the healing process. She had a hardly noticeable limp which I attributed more to her getting used to the soft cotton splint than pain. The owner was thrilled but no more than I was. She healed well and we removed the plate and screws three to four months post-op.

I was sold on the ASIF method of fracture fixation and inspired to get more advanced training in surgery and anesthesiology, preferably in a university setting. I had two partners, Drs. Gene Love and Billy Harrison, at the time and we agreed to each take time off to get further education. I would be the first to go. I chose the College of Veterinary Medicine at Colorado State University in Fort Collins, Colorado, for two main reasons: Dr. Piermattei was on the faculty and secondly, the CSU Surgical Laboratory, which at the time was arguably the best in the world. In addition, I had the option to get a Master of Science in Surgery, which I did, but that was less important to me than the additional education and training in higher level surgery and anesthesia that was offered by the Surgical Laboratory.

14

Graduate School

After my first seven years of practice experience, my surgery and anesthesia skills were average. I had limitations in both and I was honest with myself about it. I strived for optimal clinical outcome, as all veterinarians do, and some of my cases were well below that level. I wanted to get better and decided that the best way that I could improve my skills would be to get formal training in a university setting.

I chose Colorado State University because of its Surgical Laboratory, which was located on the Foothills Campus, and also because I would be able to split my time between the Lab and the Veterinary Teaching Hospital on main campus where I would be a surgery resident. I applied to Graduate School for the Master of Science in Surgery program and was accepted.

The Surgical Lab was research-oriented with experimental and "real world" cases for training in new and developing anesthesia and surgical methodology. The aortic valve stenosis repair in a dog, referred to elsewhere in this book, is an example. This was open chest surgery utilizing hypothermia in conjunction with general anesthesia. This case presented to the Veterinary Teaching Hospital on main campus and was subsequently referred to the Surgical Lab for surgery. It was certainly not an everyday case that one would expect to see in a private practice, but it was an excellent thoracic surgery teaching case.

Another example of new surgical methodology that was being developed at the Lab was a new surgical approach to intervertebral discs of the spine. This technique enabled a surgeon to access the spine using a lateral approach and provided easy entry into the lateral aspect of a disc and was primarily used to remove calcified material from a disc before it ruptured. Rupture of a calcified disc and release of calcified material into the spinal canal is painful and will cause swelling in the spinal cord that can eventually result in a loss of nerve function. A simple incision into the lateral disc wall provides an entry into the core of the disc and facilitates fairly easy removal of existing calcified material, preferably before herniation occurs, although it can also facilitate removal of calcified disc material from the spinal canal if rupture has already occured. It was considered primarily a prophylactic procedure and one that I used many times back home in practice.

Students at the Lab were extremely fortunate to be taught by three distinguished professors who were legends in their respective professional disciplines. William Lumb, DVM, MS, PhD, Dsc (hon), DACVS, DACVA, was the Director of the Lab. He taught abdominal surgery and anesthesiology. Harry Gorman, DVM, MS, DACVS, taught orthopedic surgery and bio-instrumentation. Henry Swan II, MD, Dsc (hon), FACS, former Chief of Surgery at the University of Colorado Medical Center, taught thoracic surgery. One of Dr. Swan's many claims to fame in human medicine was his development of a procedure known as "Open Chest Cardiac Massage". In addition to their teaching duties, each conducted research at the Lab.

Patricia Chase, MD, FACA, taught anesthesiology and split her time between the Surgical Lab and the teaching veterinary hospital on main campus. She was an excellent teacher who, one might speculate, preferred veterinary anesthesiology over its human counterpart. Luckily for students like myself, she ended up at CSU.

Another faculty member was Harry Ferguson, MD, FACS. Dr. Ferguson was a local head and neck surgeon in private practice who brought much practical experience in surgery of an important area that veterinary students did not receive much detailed training in at the time. At least that was my experience.

Part of the Surgical Lab curriculum was a rotation through Poudre Valley Hospital in Fort Collins, a local human hospital that served northern Colorado and southern Wyoming. For one full semester each student at the Surgical Lab would spend one day a week observing and scrubbing on surgical cases at the hospital. I participated in many of them as first assistant. In fact, one case involved an arthrodesis of the big toe because of severe osteoarthritis. The orthopedist, who was boarded certified, was shaking like a leaf in a gale, especially his hands. I never knew why but he was unable to physically perform. He asked me if I would help and I agreed to do what he thought needed to be done. I had done arthrodeses before I came to CSU, so I was not on totally unfamiliar ground, just a different species. So I worked while the orthopedist looked on. The surgery was straightforward: remove the articular cartilage inside the joint and then immobilize the joint with Kirschner wire. The fixation was solid and the joint was totally immobilized. I did not have the opportunity to follow the case but I assume that it healed well. I preferred orthopedic cases but I also worked in neurosurgery and soft tissue surgery.

I'll always remember a very competent orthopedist who I helped on several cases, including several hip replacements. I could identify him from a distance because he always wore white, high top cowboy boots with the legs of his scrub pants tucked in.

My work at Poudre Valley Hospital was a good learning experience that gave me insight into surgical techniques that were different from what I was familiar with. After arriving back home I continued to learn about different surgical techniques by assisting on cases with an orthopedist friend of mine at a local hospital in El Paso. I finished my time at Poudre Valley Hospital envious of the human surgeons because of all of the equipment and instrumentation they had immediately available to them. And, of course, they always had help, at least one and more often than not two others, depending on the procedure, scrubbed in and assisting and at least one or two available for whatever the surgeon might need. And there was always an anesthesiologist who monitored the patient from beginning to end of the procedure and, with the help of a recovery nurse, throughout the recovery period as well. In my career I probably did at least 90% of my surgeries solo, with the only help (if I was lucky) being one tech in the room with me. But, there I go again trying to compare apples and oranges.

I observed and participated in surgical techniques that I had not previously seen or used in veterinary surgery, but I was mature and experienced enough to know that I had no desire to become a human surgeon. I was perfectly happy and completely satisfied with my career as a veterinary surgeon.

Most of my surgery cases at CSU were at the Veterinary Teaching Hospital on main campus. My two primary teachers were Dr. Kenneth Smith, who was also my faculty advisor, and Dr. James Creed. Both were outstanding surgeons and I was fortunate to be able to work with them. I also worked with Dr. Piermattei but He was at the Teaching Hospital on a limited basis because he split his time between there and a surgical specialty practice in Denver.

Initially, I assisted on cases with either Dr. Smith or Dr. Creed. It didn't take long for me to gain their confidence and they pretty much turned me loose on my own. Many of my cases were routine, at least for someone who had already been in practice for seven or so years. Being a university teaching hospital we got referrals from area-wide practices, especially Denver, on a daily basis. Most of the referred cases were more difficult and less common conditions than a typical general practitioner would want to, or know how to, deal with. Many of my referral cases involved herniated intervertebral discs, often causing a partial to complete loss of nerve function in the back legs of dogs. Many of those cases were assigned to me, at least partly because of the new knowledge regarding IV disc surgery that I had just picked up at the Surgical Lab. I never intended to become a neurosurgeon, but I enjoyed the challenge and the surgery and eventually became pretty comfortable with it.

I had a case that I have never forgotten. It was a small terrier mix, middle age female in generally good health that was referred to the hospital by a local vet who had been treating her for a herniated thoracolumbar disc. I was the receiving resident when she arrived. The referring vet sent diagnosis and treatment history, which was of several days duration. His diagnosis was accurate as confirmed by our followup radiographs. The clinical neurologic signs were consistent with the history and the medical treatment that he had administered was appropriate, but she was not responding. The neurologic signs at admission into the hospital suggested minimal nerve function with minimal to absent perception of deep pain in the back legs and loss of voluntary urinary function.

The xrays showed a well-defined lesion in the spinal canal where the disc had ruptured. I explained to the owner that surgery or continuing medical treatment were both options, but with either the prognosis for a favorable outcome was guarded to poor, largely because of the extended period of time since the rupture occurred and likely irreversible damage to the spinal cord with subsequent loss of nerve function. The owner was committed and opted for surgery.

My choice for surgical procedure the next morning was a hemilaminectomy, which involves removing part of the bone of the vertebrae that surrounds the spinal cord. We exposed the spinal cord and removed considerable calcified disc material in the canal that was compressing and causing severe swelling in the spinal cord. The surgery went well and we continued with medical treatment and nursing care during hospitalization.

After several days I could see no improvement in neurologic function or deep pain perception. I advised the owner that we had done all that we could and it was my opinion that she was not going to improve. I strongly suspected that the loss of nerve function to the dog's back legs was permanent. The owner did not want to give up yet and she took her home with medication that we dispensed.

About two months later Edita and I ran into the owner at a Fort Collins restaurant. I thought to myself that the dog had probably been euthanized by now and I was dreading this conversation. The owner was thrilled to see us and she immediately started telling me about how well her dog was doing. She was happy, urinating without help, bearing weight on the back legs and walking, albeit still somewhat wobbly but still improving. She was functional and capable of taking care of herself. The owner was happy and thanked me for what I had done. I was as thrilled as she was, but I seriously doubted that what I did for the dog had much to do with its improvement. I wondered whether there might have been some divine intervention although I didn't mention that to her.

My take away from this experience: on one hand don't knowingly give "false hope" and on the other be honest with the owner but be cautious about using the word "never". Given time and natural healing ability that I believe all animals have, the body might well be capable of healing itself when sometimes we can't. I've seen it happen too many times to not believe it.

Another reason for my returning to school was to learn more about anesthesiology and Dr. Lumb's course at the Surgical Lab was in-depth and excellent. He was a great teacher in both theory and practice. He and Dr. Chase brought me up to speed on pulmonary physiology and anesthesiology pretty quickly.

In the late '60's and early '70's, prior to my time at CSU, I frequently saw cases of hip dysplasia mainly in larger dogs for which there was no reliable physical correction. Hip dysplasia is essentially a ball and socket joint in which the head of the femur (ball) luxates in and out of the acetabulum (socket). It's painful and eventually develops into osteoarthritis, which causes a lifetime of pain and dysfunction. About the best that we could hope for at the time was long-term pain medication which often had serious side effects.

Around 1970, I had a client with a St. Bernard that, at the age of about one year, was already showing signs of painful hip dysplasia. Radiography showed mild looseness in one hip and subluxation in the other. I offered to refer them to CSU or Texas A&M for a consult and possible surgery but because money was an issue they declined. I offered, at no cost to the owner, to try a technique that I had not performed but that I believed had promise. They accepted.

The surgery was relatively simple. I applied a strip of teflon over the upper rim of the socket in a way that would extend, or overhang, the rim enough to prevent the ball from luxating or migrating out of the socket. I anchored the strip with several bone screws. Theoretically, given the dog's young age and probability for continuing musculoskeletal development, if I could prevent the ball from luxating out of the socket, that might allow the muscles and ligamentous tissue surrounding the hip to tighten in a way that would keep the ball more deeply seated into the socket.

The outcome was less beneficial than I hoped for, partly because limiting the young dog's activity was difficult. He did show improvement for a few weeks post-op which I attributed to pain medicine. But as we began to reduce the dose, the pain increased and lameness in that leg became increasingly intense. An x-ray at one month post-op showed that the screws had loosened, the teflon strip was showing signs of wear and tear and the hip was beginning to subluxate. This experience was frustrating and all I could do was just keep hoping that someone would come up with a good solution to the problem.

There were a lot of researchers who were working to develop a reliable hip prosthesis and the hope was that a better one for animals might lead to a better one for humans. Dr. Gorman was at the forefront of this work and developed the first total hip joint replacement for dogs in the late fifties. It was less than desirable and its use was short-lived. He continued his research at the Surgical Lab and I was privileged to sit in on some of his presentations regarding his progress. Another reason that I was glad to be at CSU.

I was technically considered a surgery resident and graduate student and I also worked as an instructor at times with third and fourth year students, interns and other residents. I enjoyed the time I spent with them in surgery and sharing with them my seven years of private practice experience. Most of them intended to eventually go into private practice and were anxious to learn more about it. On the other hand it gave me an opportunity to learn from them about the latest in diagnostic and therapeutic methods and technology.

My time at CSU was every bit as good as I had hoped it would be. I completed my Masters and Edita and I returned to El Paso in August, 1973, anxious to share new knowledge and enthusiasm with clients and their animals.

After arriving back in El Paso I seriously considered changing from general practice to a small animal surgery specialty practice. That was in the early 1970's when private specialty practice and board certification were still fairly new concepts in veterinary medicine. I did have the Masters degree which was proof of formal training in a specialty. In a specialty practice I would depend on referrals from the immediate area, which would include southern New Mexico and far West Texas and would have to make a substantial investment in new surgical and anesthetic monitoring equipment, radiography, ultrasound, etc. El Paso was still a fairly small city, but it was growing and my practice had excellent growth potential, but only as a general small animal practice. I finally decided that there would not be enough referral work to justify the expense of gearing up for specialization and I canned the idea.

After the word spread that I was back with a Masters in Surgery I did, however, begin to get referrals from El Paso and the surrounding area. Not a lot but enough to keep up my interest and use the training I had just worked hard to get. There were simply not enough vets in El Paso and surrounding communities to expect to make a living in a referral surgical specialty practice. So, I continued as a general predominantly small animal practice with some large animal work which was mostly back yard type horses.

15

Field Surgery

We were hunting bobwhite quail and pheasant fifteen or so miles southwest of Arkansas City, Kansas, just north of the Oklahoma state line. I was with Don, a long-time upland bird hunting friend, and his dogs Daisy and Molly. We were walking a field that belonged to Marty, another long-time friend who farmed and raised cattle in the area and lived a few miles from where we were hunting.

It was not a huge field by any means, perhaps a hundred or so acres, but it's knee-high stand of grass provided good cover for birds. The grain fields on two sides made for easy access to food and the small drainage that ran from east to west through the property always held water. It was really good habitat for birds. We hunted this field on previous trips and always moved both bobwhite quail and pheasant. It was surrounded by a 4-strand barbed wire fence. Marty would occasionally run cattle on it but there weren't any present on this trip. It was a small, easily-hunted field compared to most that we hunt, and since it was late morning we decided to knock it out in an hour or two and then head into Ark City for lunch at Daisy Mae's cafe, after which Don's dog Daisy was named. Don decided to take Molly, the older of the two dogs, for some exercise and fun. Both dogs were Labradors, Molly was black and Daisy was blonde. Molly was 11 or 12 years old at the time and was showing early signs of arthritis which limited how long and hard she could or would want to hunt. But she would always put her heart into it and do her best to find birds for us.

We didn't find the quail that we normally do on that ground but we did move a few pheasant and Molly was obviously enjoying herself. We were a hundred or so yards apart when Don yelled at me. I looked up and he was kneeling on the ground next to Molly. I walked over and Molly's left front leg was covered with blood from her elbow down to her toes. She was standing and bearing weight on it, which was a relief, but she had a nasty laceration on the front side of her elbow. It was a vertical, 4" to 5" laceration, U-shaped and located over the front of her elbow. From side to side it was 3" to 4" and the skin was separated from the underlying tissue all the way up the leg to just above the bend of the elbow. There appeared to be minimal injury to the underlying muscle but none to nerves, significant arteries or veins. She continued to bleed, not gushing but a steady drip.

As she was covering ground in front of Don in grass that was just deep enough to limit her visibility, she ran through the fence and obviously engaged some barbs. Fortunately, we had already made the turn at the south end of the field and were headed north where the truck was parked about a half mile away. We didn't have anything that we could use to stop the bleeding and she could walk okay so we just double-timed it to the truck which took only a few minutes.

We dropped the tailgate and put Molly on it to get a better look at the wound. It had to hurt like heck but she showed no sign of pain. After a good look I confirmed my initial suspicion that there was no serious damage done to any major arteries, veins or nerves. The muscle had a few nicks which was the main source of the continued bleeding and needed to be closed with sutures. The wound needed to be cleaned and the skin flap reattached to the underlying muscle as soon as possible to give the circulation a chance to reestablish it's flow to the skin in order to prevent loss of part or possibly all of the skin flap. I was pretty sure that she would lose part of the skin around the edge of the flap, which would be no big deal, but if she lost the entire flap it would take forever for the wound to heal and probably leave a large scar that might interfere with her elbow function. Now we had to make a decision.

We had two options: she needed surgery as soon as possible, so we could either take her into Arkansas City and hopefully find a clinic that could get to her quickly because of the circulation, or lack thereof, issue which I speculated might require a general anesthetic and, if so, perhaps an overnight stay in the clinic, or we could repair it immediately where we were. Our plan was to leave the next morning for Pratt, Kansas, which was about a 3 hour drive west of Arkansas City via Wichita where we wanted to visit a Cabela's store to pick up some supplies and then on to Pratt to hook up with an outfitter for a couple days of guided bird hunting.

The advantage of taking her to an Ark City clinic was that the surgery would be done in a much cleaner environment. The hair over and around the laceration could be clipped and the wound could probably be cleaned more effectively. The disadvantage was that we would have no control over how soon the surgery could be done. She might sit in a cage for a couple of hours before they could get to her, almost guaranteeing that there would be at least some skin lost from the flap.

The advantage of doing the surgery where we were was that it could be done right here and now. All we had to do was numb the area with a local anesthetic and get to work. This would give us a better chance to save as much of the skin flap as possible. A less important advantage, but nevertheless a consideration, was that it would probably cost several hundred dollars at a clinic compared to zero if we did it.

We discussed the matter for a few minutes and decided that, all things considered, we should go ahead and do it on the spot as I pulled out my medicine bag from the back of the pickup.

Hunting dogs are always getting scrapes, minor cuts or, as in Molly's case, severe lacerations, snake bites or worse. They chase birds into mesquite bushes, prickly pears or other vegetation that the birds deem to be good cover, sometimes forgetting to close their eyes, often resulting in eyelid or corneal abrasions, lacerations, thorns, stickers from cactus, etc. And then there are the all too common wrestling matches with porcupines and skunks. For these reasons I always carry a medicine bag stocked with a good supply of medications, such as eye and skin antibiotic ointments, a myriad of bandage supplies, syringes and needles, pain medication and sedative, injectable steroids and antibiotics, medications for upset gastrointestinal tracts, betadine wound scrub and cleaner and sterile saline solution for rinsing a wound, sterile surgery drapes, sterile surgery gloves and a sterile surgery pack suitable for most trauma surgeries, such as Molly's. In the desert southwest where we mostly hunt, extended hunts on hot days sometimes cause dehydration, so I also carry intravenous catheters, infusion sets and fluids just in case.

We parked the truck in a position that provided the most direct sunlight for best visibility of the wound and then we placed Molly on the tailgate with her left side up. She was completely cooperative until I began to inject the wound with the local anesthetic. She did not like that at all and wasn't timid about telling us so. I couldn't blame her. I don't like it either when I have to get a local, but after the burning pain subsided she would feel no more pain throughout the procedure. In fact the only time she complained about being held down after the local was when she just got tired of being restrained. Her cooperation made the entire process so much faster and easier and enabled me to do a better job. If she had not been so easy to work with she would have needed at least a sedative and probably a general anesthetic which definitely would have required a trip to an Ark City clinic.

The next step was to clean the wound and area immediately around it using betadine surgical scrub soap and sterile saline. I spent at least ten to fifteen minutes scrubbing, rinsing, scrubbing, rinsing, etc., etc., until all of the dirt, weed seeds, dried blood and anything else that looked like it didn't belong there was removed. This was a critical part of the entire process because if the wound was going to heal the way I hoped it would, we had to start with a wound as clean as we could possibly make it. After the last rinse I painted the wound and surrounding skin with betadine solution, applied the sterile drape and put on sterile gloves and began to remove non-viable tissue from the entire length and on both sides of the wound. I trimmed the skin at the edge of the flap to shape it a bit and remove all tissue that had lost its blood supply. To get into healthy bleeding tissue it was necessary to remove a considerable amount of the edge of the flap and the opposite skin edge which would place tension on the sutures and suture line, especially when Molly would extend her elbow. The practical effect of this would be to cause the sutures to cut through the edge of the flap and allow the suture line to open, thereby delaying healing. To prevent that possibility I separated the skin at the upper part of the flap from the underlying muscle using blunt dissection scissors and left just enough slack in it to keep tension from becoming an issue.

I closed a few superficial cuts in the muscle with sutures and then placed two small drain tubes, one on either side of the wound, entering through two small skin incisions above and exiting through two incisions below it. The purpose of the tubes was to allow the wound to drain blood, serum or purulent discharge if infection occurred, which frankly I thought was highly probable.

Before suturing the wound closed I applied an antibiotic solution liberally to help to prevent infection. Sutures pulled the two sides of the wound together nicely with no obvious tension. Then I placed several sutures to eliminate the "dead" space between skin and muscle caused by the nature of the laceration and my blunt dissection. Overall, the closure looked good and if we could prevent or at least minimize infection it had a good chance to heal by "first intention". The entire procedure took about an hour and a half, only because Molly was so agreeable and easy to work with.

After applying a comfortable cotton bandage from the tip of her toes to well above her elbow, we were finished. After an antibiotic injection and some pain medicine we loaded Molly in her kennel, gave her water and a treat and drove to Ark City for lunch at Daisy Mae's cafe.

We met Marty and his coffee buddies at Daisy Mae's at six the next morning. Just sitting and listening to the conversation among those local ranchers and farmers has always been worth the trip there. After breakfast and a good visit we made a swing by the local donut shop to pick up donuts, sweet rolls and coffee to snack on while driving and then we got on the road. We were in Pratt early that afternoon and decided to give the dogs and ourselves the rest of the day to relax and get ready to hunt the following day.

Our first day of hunting went well. There were plenty of quail and pheasant to keep us and Daisy (of course we didn't hunt Molly) busy and happy. We checked Molly's wound after lunch. The suture line showed a slight blood-tinged watery discharge. I had given her an injectable antibiotic daily since the incident, mainly because I had forgotten to pack cephalexin, my go-to antibiotic for injuries such as hers. Even though I wasn't yet worried about the discharge, I decided that she should be on cephalexin, so we drove back to a drug store in Pratt that I had noticed as we left town that morning. The pharmacist gladly filled my prescription order for a two week supply and I started Molly as soon as we got back to the truck. We resumed hunting that afternoon and ended up having a good day.

We changed the bandage daily for several days to keep it clean and discourage Molly's licking (unfortunately we didn't have an e-collar with us). I also wanted to keep a little compression on the wound to encourage redevelopment of circulation in the skin flap.

We were back home in El Paso after another day of hunting and the thin discharge from the suture line was diminishing. The skin was soft and warm to the touch, suggesting a good blood supply and no sign of infection. We left her unwrapped but kept an e-collar on to be sure she didn't lick. I removed the drain tubes at 5 days post-op and began to remove a few sutures every day or so until they were all out by 14 days. The wound would not have healed any better even if it had been done in an operating room environment.

Happily, Molly went on to enjoy life for a few more years and many more bird hunts. She never lost her enthusiasm. We are left with many good memories of her.

16

Honey, Trike and Judy

She hobbled into my exam room on three legs that morning led by a volunteer for the local animal rescue league after she had been found on the side of a road in the upper valley. I picked her up off the floor and put her on the exam table. She sat there like a statue, not making a move and wondering what would happen next. She made no effort to get off the table or resist us in any way. It didn't take a genius to quickly realize that her short life had not been easy.

She was a Border Collie, about a year old, orange and white, and a little on the thin side. She was scruffy and looked as if she'd never had a bath. By the looks of her mammary glands she had recently been nursing pups. She had no collar, tag, tattoo or implanted microchip or anything else that would identify her. Her vital signs were normal although, along with being thin, she appeared to be mildly anemic which I suspected was caused by lack of food, nursing pups and possibly intestinal parasites.

Her right front foot was displaced laterally from her carpal joint down to the tips of her toes, at about a 45 degree angle to her fore-leg. There were no obvious palpable fractures and only the slightest movement in the carpus when I manipulated it. It was almost a com-pletely frozen joint. Cutaneous nerve function and pain perception were present from her car-pus down to her toes. I did a physical exam and, pain or discomfort notwithstanding, she never objected. In a word, she was "stoic". She had a look in her eyes that told me she really wanted help, but had just about given up on ever getting any.

The volunteer would foster her until she was healthy enough to be adopted, assuming, in the unlikely scenario that they could find someone who would be willing to adopt a lame dog that was likely going to stay that way for the rest of her life. My guess was that she had been down on her luck for most of her life and was about ready to throw in the towel. Nothing that might happen to her while in my care now would come close to what she had already been through no doubt many times.

Later that day we radiographed the leg and ruled out a fracture of the carpals, metacarpals or toes. The heavy ligamentous tissue (joint capsule) that wrapped around the carpus had been been torn on the inner part of the joint. The loss of stabilization and her attempts to bear weight on the joint eventually led to the lateral deviation. The carpus was now filled with dense, fibrinous material, suggesting that she had been living with the pain and disuse of the leg for probably at least a couple of months. The flexor tendons between the carpus and toes were contracted from disuse and as a result her toes were severely contracted.

I advised the rescue league that there was a good chance that we could straighten the leg but to the extent that it would be functional and pain-free, only time would tell. The prognosis for a pain-free leg was guarded. If we failed to get a good outcome from the first procedure, we could come back later and surgically arthrodese (fuse) the joint. If that failed and she continued to have pain, we could amputate the leg. Admirably, the rescue league agreed to try so we kept her in the clinic with plans for surgery the next day.

We drew blood for a preanesthetic chemistry and blood count. The only test that was outside normal limits was her red blood cell count which was only slightly below normal. Her fecal and heartworm tests were negative. After microchipping and vaccinating her we put her in a cage with food and water. We could tell that she was hungry and probably thirsty too but she didn't trust us. Her eyes shifted from us to the food and back to us. She needed food and water so we walked out of the room and left her alone. I checked on her about an hour later and the food was gone, as was about half the water. She sat up and looked at me as if to wonder whether she had done something wrong and whether or not she would punished....again.

That evening she ate all of the food we gave her, which we limited since she would go to surgery the next morning. Her appetite was a good sign. By now, my staff was beginning to like this dog and so was I. Lots of patting, rubbing her head and belly and being talked to was very therapeutic. Exactly what she needed and wanted. We were very slowly overcoming her distrust.

We started an intravenous drip and administered a preanesthetic sedative. When she was sedate, we gave her an ultra-short acting iv anesthetic called propoflo to induce general anesthesia to the level that we could place a tube down her trachea. We then hooked her up to our anesthetic machine which flowed a gas anesthetic/oxygen mixture. Knowing that this would be a painful, but not necessarily long procedure (I was planning on about thirty minutes surgery time), I told my tech, who was monitoring her ecg, pulse rate and blood oxygen level, to keep her deep until I was finished with my physical manipulation.

The manipulation went well. No incisions required, physical manipulation only. It was a matter of breaking down the fibrinous adhesions inside the carpal joint. It was critical to do so without making things worse, i.e., fracturing one or more carpal bones or perhaps a meta-carpal, or damaging a blood vessel or nerve. We were able to eliminate the adhesions to the extent that she had a range of motion much closer to normal. I applied a Robert Jones splint (a comfortable cotton splint that most dogs tolerate well) from just above the elbow down to just below the toes. I gave her an injection of pain medicine before she was awake for some relief from the pain that I knew she would have. She quickly recovered from the anesthetic and rested well in her cage. We offered her a light meal later in the day.

The following morning she actually wagged her tail just a bit when I walked into the cage room to check on her. I was starting to believe that she knew that we were helping her. She had not touched the splint overnight and was bright and alert. She ate a good breakfast. The volunteer came for her later in the day and I noticed another slight tail wag. Another good sign. We sent her home with pain medicine and instructions to limit her activity and see her back in three days.

At the three day checkup she was still re-served but we all agreed that she was a little more outgoing and maybe a bit happy to see us. She might have remembered all the belly rubs she got while she was here. The splint was clean and dry and holding well.

The volunteer told us that she was unable to keep the dog any longer and the rescue league was looking for another foster to take her in while she continued to heal. She also said that the league was hoping to adopt her out soon because they were short on space. She had not been adopted yet probably because she had not been at the league location where the ani-mals are viewed and adoptions take place. The volunteer added that as well-behaved as she was and because she was young, she would probably adopt out quickly. But then again, it might not be easy to find someone who would be willing to pick up the expense of further treatment for her leg, if that became necessary.

The volunteer agreed to let the league know that we needed her back in a week, but before leaving she asked if any of us had an idea of a good name for her. Edita was standing nearby and immediately volunteered, "She's a honey of a dog, so how about naming her Honey?" That was it. The name stuck. She was now and forever would be "Honey". It was a perfect name for her.

Edita and I had been without a dog for some time and we had already discussed adopting Honey. She called the league headquarters and told them we'd love to take her home with us. They agreed, we signed the adoption papers, returned all of the fee that the league had paid us for the care that we had given her and Honey had a new home and family. She absolutely adored our three kids and they loved her back. For the next thirteen years she was truly a "member of our family".

Her leg healed as well as I had hoped for with splinting only. The carpal joint redeveloped very dense adhesions which essentially immobilized the joint the way it was when I first saw her, except now it was better aligned with no lateral deviation. As she began to bear weight, the contracted tendons began to lengthen enough for her to be able to slightly extend her foot. Her foot and toe joints from her carpus down were ankylosed, or frozen, which minimized movement in the joints, which in turn minimized pain.

She would occasionally get a little gimpy on the leg but a couple days of pain medications would always take care of it. All in all, the leg condition was never much of a factor in her life.

I had some smart dogs in my life but Honey was by far the most intelligent. Shortly after we brought her home for the first time, she had a bowel movement in the living room. Edita saw her do it and firmly told her "no". That's all Honey needed to hear. In all the years we had her, and she spent a lot of time inside with us, she never did it again. She would simply go to the back door and stand there until we would let her out.

Border Collies are herding dogs and so was Honey. We have a four feet high rock/wrought iron wall that encloses our backyard and separates it from a sharp drop-off onto a steep slope covered with cactus, mesquite and other desert vegetation. When my oldest grandson, Jack, was still a toddler he would play around in the back yard and Honey would always keep a close eye on him. If he got within about five feet or so from the wall she would trot over to him, get between him and the wall and start to direct him away from it by bumping her nose against his little diaper-covered bottom. When she had him where she knew he was safe, she'd lie down, but continue to watch him. Whenever he would head back toward the wall, she'd jump up and go back into her toddler-herding mode. She was absolutely not going to let that kid get too close to the wall.

Once I was working in the back yard and not paying attention to Honey who was with me. I left the side gate open and she started to explore and left the yard thru the gate. When I was finished, I looked for her and she was nowhere to be seen. I went back into the house and told Edita that Honey had gotten out and was gone. The search was on. We rechecked the back yard, checked the front yard, up and down the street...no Honey. I went back into the house and opened the front door. There she was sitting as close to the door as she could possibly get. She could not get back into the house fast enough. She was ecstatic about being back where she wanted to be, as evidenced by her running in circles and standing straight up on her back legs and spinning round and round in one place. It was obvious that she was not anxious to be a homeless dog again. She had been there, done that and did not wish to repeat it.

Another long-time member of our family arrived at our clinic in a way that was similar to that of Honey. A traveling salesman who was passing through the city enroute to the west coast saw the cat near the service station just off the interstate where he stopped for gas. She was walking on three legs with the fourth one dangling. He was able to get her into his car and then, following the directions of the station attendant, drove straight to our clinic which was only a short drive.

She was a calico domestic long-hair, about six months old and, except for her front leg issue, was in generally good shape. She had no collar, tag, chip, tattoo or any means of identification. Her vital signs were normal. Just like Honey, she was obviously fearful but did not resist my exam. She was so easy to work with that I was certain that she wasn't feral. We speculated that she probably had a home but was either allowed to go outside or perhaps escaped from the house and was hit by a car.

I advised the salesman, whose name I regretfully have long since forgotten but who I will always remember, that I would have to x-ray the fracture before I would know for sure what needed to be done to repair it. In addition, I would need to do some blood testing to more fully evaluate her health. He said that he would love to give her a home but because of his travels he would not be able to keep her. In fact, he had to be in Phoenix that night. He asked if we would take care of her, do everything necessary to restore her to good health, and then try to find her owner. We agreed to do just that. Then, and this really blew us away, he said he wanted to pay for whatever was needed to get her back to normal. He never asked how much it was going to cost, he simply pulled out his wallet and credit card, laid them on the exam table and asked which we preferred.

Over the course of my entire career I have known and worked for some good people who genuinely loved animals and would do absolutely anything for them. This man's generosity was a bit overwhelming. He was one of the best.

After thanking him for his dedication to this little stray cat that he had only known for about an hour, I agreed to do whatever was necessary to bring her back to good health and assured him that if we were unable to find her owner, we would find a good home for her. Then, I declined his payment. He insisted, but I held firm. He thanked us for what we did, gave her a few nice pats and was out the front door and off to Phoenix.

About a week later he called and asked how she was doing. We gave him a progress report and told him all was well. He was pleased. We never heard from him again. He was truly a good Samaritan.

Her xray revealed a mid-shaft, transverse fracture of the radius and ulna. It was a clean fracture with very little splintering. It was the type of fracture that would probably heal very well with a splint, especially considering her young age, but at that time we had no idea where she might end up as an adoptee or whether we would be able to follow up for an occasional xray and splint change, I opted for surgery, which would give her a much better chance to heal properly even if she did not get the recommended exams. All of her blood tests were normal, so we applied a temporary splint and set her up for surgery in two days to give her a chance to become somewhat acclimated to her surroundings and to get a few good meals.

Another concern was the possibility of damage to the radial nerve which is fairly common with that type of fracture and its location. But, fracture repair was first priority and about all we could do, if in fact the nerve was damaged, would be to give it time to heal.

The surgery went well. I was able to get two small pins into the full length of the medullary canal of the radius. The alignment of the radius and ulna and apposition at the fracture site appeared to be good visually, but we confirmed that, as we always do after fracture repair, with xrays. She recovered uneventfully and we kept her in the clinic for a couple more days.

In the meantime Edita placed an ad in the local newspaper's "lost and found" section which ran for about a month. We never got any response to it. She also called Animal Control daily to see if anyone had reported her missing. No luck there either. We weren't worried about getting her into a good home because we had many clients who we knew well that we were sure would take her.

After a couple days recovering in the clinic we decided to take her home with us to get her into a little more relaxed environment. This would also give us more time to follow up on the surgery and any further treatment that might be necessary. (By now I suspect that most readers know where this story is going). The longer we had her, the more attached we were to her and the less effort we put into getting her into a good home. We decided that if anyone stepped up and claimed her as their own, we would certainly let her go. Otherwise, she would become a permanent member of our family.

After a couple of months the fracture was completely healed and I removed the pins. It soon became obvious that the injured nerve had not healed to the extent that it was functional and capable of properly bearing weight. If not corrected she would have a lifetime of never-ending ulcerations on the top of her foot caused by knuckling over of her foot at the carpal joint, and an atrophied, essentially useless limb. In my experience amputation was the best, long-term correction for that problem and that is what I chose to do. The surgery went well and she recovered uneventfully. She was already accustomed to using three legs so she hardly noticed the absence of the fourth.

Up to that time we had not named her, but what better name for a three-legged cat than "Tricycle", or, "Trike" for short. She now had an official name.

Trike loved to go outside and we would occasionally let her out into the back yard, but only if one of us could keep an eye on her to be sure she didn't take off. She would hide under bushes and watch birds fly into and over the yard. One day there was a lot of dove activity in the yard so she slowly crept her way from the bush she had been hidden in out onto the grass and got as flat on her belly as she could and assumed her "ambush" position. One bird came flying into the yard obviously intending to land on the grass. Trike and the bird saw each other at the same instant, the bird aborted the landing and started flying hard to gain altitude before it reached Trike, and when it was directly over her she jumped straight up about 4 feet, swatted at it with her one front leg, whacked it good and knocked it down. It was not injured but was stunned for a second before it jumped up and flew off. Trike had a look on her face as if to say "who needs four legs?"

She was twelve years old when one day she somehow found her way out of the house. We noticed her absence shortly after she went missing and immediately went into an all-out search mode. We thoroughly searched our house and front and back yards those of our nearby neighbors. She was nowhere to be found. We placed ads in the lost pet section of the newspaper, put posters up around the neighborhood, called animal control daily, knocked on doors, all to no avail. After three weeks we had all but given up on ever finding her. Edita and I attended at a funeral one day and when we returned home her mother, who was taking care of the kids while we were gone, said that we had gotten a phone call from someone saying that they thought they might have our cat. We immediately returned the call and sure enough their description sounded like Trike. It was her and she had traveled about a mile from our house. They had found her hiding under a bush in their yard.

She was thin and a little dehydrated but otherwise in good condition. We never figured out how she got there or stayed alive for three weeks. But she did. It was miraculous. She was glad to see us and even more so to see the inside of her home. She was more affectionate than usual for a couple of days but then gradually reverted back into her typically independent mode.

She helped us raise three kids and made the trip to Colorado State University with us. She was tough, durable and friendly, but only when it was her idea. She went on to live to be eighteen years old and except for the three weeks she was missing, she was a healthy, happy member of our family.

So when someone refers to their pet as a member of their family, don't laugh. It's true. Honey and Trike were a real joy to have in our family for so many years.

Another member of our family, in this case "extended" family, who certainly deserves at least a mention, if not a book (which might be my next project), was Judy, who we met on a Kansas hunt. I was with Don and Randolph, two long-time friends and hunting buddies, and we had rented an old farm house near Fellsburg, about fifteen miles north of Greensburg, for a few days of pheasant and quail hunting. It was nearly dark as we pulled into the dirt driveway after a long day of driving and as we began to unload the truck we could see movement in the old southerly-leaning garage at the end of the driveway. We could see a head peeking around the frame of the door to look at us, but every time one of us would make the slightest move in her direction, it would draw back behind the wall as if to hide. We first thought that it was a coyote, but that critter would have been long gone by now. It was a dog, wanting to see us but not wanting to be seen by us.

Figuring that she was a local dog that lived in the immediate area, we ignored her while we went on unloading the truck. But each time that we would wander back outside she would have moved a little further out of the garage and then duck back into it if we tried to approach her. She was quite thin and looked as if she had not been eating much, if any, recently. We heated and shredded a couple of flour tortillas and put them in a bowl along with a bowl of water and put both in the garage for her. While inside the garage we looked around for any evidence that someone was feeding or providing water or a bed for her to get off the cold ground. There was none. It was already cold and would probably dip well below freezing overnight and the garage provided only a wind break. We thought, "this doesn't look like a place where one would expect to find a local dog". While we speculated on how she got there, whether she was lost or abandoned or what, she kept plenty of distance between us and her, but as we walked back toward the house she jumped on the tortillas and finished that in a minute or so and then she finished off the water, probably the first food and water she'd had in days.

Next morning she was still there, standing in the doorway of the garage looking at the back door of the house, as if she was wondering whether we'd be back. We were, but this time with heated chopped meat added to the tortillas and a bigger bowl of water. After she finished that, again within minutes, she stood outside the garage looking at the back door of the house, seemingly waiting for us to return.

For a warmup hunt for us and the dogs that morning we decided to hunt a small grass field that was a short walk from the house. We geared up and with Don's two labradors started walking toward the field. About halfway there we looked back and there she was, following us but still keeping her distance. It was as if she wanted to get to know us better but still didn't trust us. She obviously was afraid of us and we were starting to think that she had been abused, abandoned or something unusual. She had a collar on but we had not been able to get close enough to examine it for personal information. She followed us while we hunted and acted like she had done that before, although she spent most of her time watching us and Don's dogs. From a distance I guessed her to be a couple years old.

When we returned to the farmhouse for lunch, she followed us back to the garage. We gave her a little more food and filled her water bowl. The farmer who owned the house we were in came around while we were having lunch. We asked him about the dog in the garage and he told us that an out-of-state outfitter had been there hunting with clients the week before we got there. He said the dog had suddenly appeared alone as soon as the outfitter had left to go back home. She had pretty much stayed in the old garage but he had seen her wandering around his place which was about a quarter mile away. He assumed that she belonged to the outfitter and had been left, intentionally or otherwise. He was pretty adamant about one thing: he did not want her on his property. He had chickens that freely roamed his yard and other livestock around his house. My impression was if he caught her showing any interest in his animals, she would be dispatched quite rapidly. On the other hand, he said that he doubted she'd be a problem for long because of all the coyotes in the area that no doubt would finish her off sooner than later. Well, now we knew for sure that she was not a local dog and that she was "between a rock and a hard place", as they say.

We speculated about how she got there but she looked and behaved like a bird dog. She was an English Pointer, liver and white in color and the collar she was wearing was blaze orange, a popular, highly visible color for hunting dogs and hunters.

Her days were numbered. We hunted in the area for three to four days and she was always in the garage waiting for us whenever we'd pull back into the driveway. She had warmed up to us a lot, mainly because of the food we gave her. We were gaining her trust, a little at a time. Finally she allowed us to get close enough to touch and pat her and from that point on she followed us around like a puppy looking for attention, and more food. Information on her collar confirmed that she belonged to the outfitter and her name was Judy. But, it was clear that regardless of who she belonged to, she wasn't going to last long unless someone assumed responsibility for her, and soon. The more we thought about her situation, i.e., being caught between a pack of coyotes and the business end of a gun, and her short life-expectancy, the more we became attached to her.

We talked about what we could do with her and after considering all options that we could think of we decided to take her home with us. We had no idea if Greensburg or Pratt, a town about 20 miles east of Greensburg, had a humane society or animal rescue organization and leaving her there to die in short order was not an option. Back home we would contact the outfitter and offer to ship Judy to him at our expense. If he didn't want her we could send her to the Humane Society of El Paso or one of the many rescue organizations locally. For Judy's safety, that seemed to be the smartest decision. Besides, we were liking her more every day.

We arrived back home a couple days later and Randolph and his wife, Sandy, agreed to keep Judy until I was able to contact the outfitter, which I did the next day. I called the phone number on the collar and he answered. I introduced myself and happily announced that we had found his dog that he had lost while in Kansas. I told him about how we had finally gained her trust and decided to bring her home with us for her safety and that we were prepared to ship her to him and would do so at our expense. He kindly thanked me for the offer but was essentially non-commital about getting her back at all. Finally, he said that if we wanted her, we could keep her.

Fortunately for Judy, she spent the rest of her life living with Randolph and Sandy and could not have had a better home. Edita and I took care of her medical needs, which early on were significant. She had heartworms, more than one kind of intestinal parasite and she was covered with fleas and a few ticks. When we finally eliminated all of those issues we spayed her and sure enough she had a moderate-grade infection in her uterus that would have only gotten worse.

In retrospect, I don't know who was luckier, Judy or those of us who lived with her. She had a unique personality with enough idiosyncracies and quirks to fill the pages of a good sized book, but we all enjoyed her as much as she did us for several more years. She made many bird hunts and had as much fun as any of us. She admittedly was not a great bird dog. She knew why we were there and what we were hunting but she was so easily distracted she would occasionally forget. She would move at a pretty good pace for a while and then for no apparent reason she would get on top of a ridge and stop and stare at the other dogs and hunters. I often wondered what she was thinking during those times. It was as if she just zoned out for a few minutes and then suddenly she would return to real time and remember where she was and what she was supposed to be doing.

One day she was a bird dog and the next a lap dog, when all she wanted was a head and ear scratch or a belly scratch, and if you would give her the slightest bit of encouragement she'd do her best to crawl up into your lap. She was persistent, she'd bug you until she was sure you knew she was there waiting for your attention. I'm certain she is not the first English Pointer that has ever shown that kind of behavior, but based on my experience with the breed, it's not typical.

Judy was always at her best as a bird dog when Randolph and I hunted alone with her. With no one else around to distract her, she was pretty good, more like one would expect with an English Pointer. She would get wind of quail, point and hold till we got to her. We would walk around and kick bushes in the direction in which she was pointing and eventually the bird or birds would flush. If we got lucky and knocked one down she would pick it up and bring it back to us....some of the time but not every time. Other times she would find the downed bird and stand over it with the "zoned out" look on her face as if she was wondering what she should do now. She always kept us guessing what she would do next. But she was predictably a better hunter when she was the only dog and Randolph and I were the only hunters. Judy was the Jekyll and Hyde of English Pointers.

We got separated from Judy one day while hunting in a near gale force wind in southern New Mexico. We were hunting on the down-wind side of a mountain in a steady westerly wind of about 20 to 30 mph with frequent gusts up to 40 and higher. Walking was difficult and hearing was even more so. Judy was hunting 30 to 40 yards ahead of us and she would occasionally look back to see where we were. Then she'd take off again. The only control we had over her was vocal. When she'd get too far out ahead of us we'd yell at her to get her attention and she would either return to us or wait for us to catch up with her. The gusting wind started to kick up dust and literally made it impossible to hear what someone standing only a few feet away would say. The conditions became unhuntable so we decided to head back to the truck. But, where was Judy?

We stood still for a few minutes looking at all of the draws and arroyos and ridges around us hoping to catch a glimpse of her. No Judy. There were several other hunters with us that day and we all split up and walked in differ-ent directions yelling her name and looking for tracks that we thought might be hers. No Judy. We finally decided that she was probably un-able to hear us and became disoriented while she was looking for us. We forgot about hunt-ing and went into a search and rescue mode for several hours and made no contact with her.

We walked back to the trucks hoping that she had found her way back to them. But she wasn't there either. After a quick lunch we started walking again with our shotguns just in case we bumped up some quail, but we were mostly looking for Judy. We all knew what she faced if were didn't find her. Odds were she wouldn't last more than a day or so, pretty much the same situation she was in when we first found her. She had no food or water and would be surrounded by coyotes and possibly a mountain lion or two. She wouldn't last long. There was a chance she would be seen and picked up by another hunter in the area who would then hopefully contact us at our phone number on her collar. We wouldn't say it but none of us held out much hope that we'd ever see her again.

We were spread out over about a quarter mile area just north of where we last saw Judy. It was mid-afternoon, the wind was still blowing but not quite as gusty as earlier in the day and we were in the middle of a good-sized covey and getting an occasional shot when someone starting yelling "there's Judy, there's Judy", and was pointing downhill. We looked down and sure enough there she was a couple hundred yards downhill trotting directly toward us in the same arroyo we were in. Obviously she saw us and couldn't get to us fast enough. Nor could we get to her fast enough. It was a joyful reunion.

Except for being mildly dehydrated she was in good physical condition. She was so thirsty we had to give her small portions of water to keep her from overdrinking and throwing it all back up. She was exhausted. As happy as she was she didn't want to stand for very long at a time. We let her just sit and catch her breath for a half hour or so and continued with small drinks of water to rehydrate her. Someone had a candy bar and gave her half of it which she inhaled. A while later he gave her the other half and by then she was feeling better and showing more signs of excited happiness now that she was back with her friends.

We walked slowly with her back to the trucks which were only about a quarter mile away. She showed no inclination to separate herself from us. In fact she stayed as close to us as she could get.

We finally decided that she wandered downhill from the point that we last saw her and eventually found the dirt road that we had entered the area on. It ran north and south and when she cut the road she had to make a decision...go left or go right. A right hand turn would have taken her into more isolated country and lowered the chance that she might have seen us or someone else who might have rescued her. Fortunately she took a left hand turn and headed in a northerly direction which eventually would have gotten her out of the hunting area and into a more civilized area with an occasional residence where she might have gotten help, assuming she lived long enough.

The dirt road took her in a direction that put her about a quarter mile directly below us and the wind direction was perfect to carry to her the sound of a couple of shots we made. She was familiar with shotguns and recognized the sounds as shots. She probably thought "where there are shots there must be people", so she turned uphill and headed toward the shot reports. The rising quail, shots and wind saved her life.

Several years later Judy developed a blood-tinged nasal discharge that I suspected might be an abcessed tooth or perhaps a sinus infection. There was no visible pathology in her mouth but I decided to treat her symptomatically with antibiotic and a low-dose steroid. A couple weeks later the discharge persisted and swelling was developing in her eye. We biopsied her nasal sinus and the diagnosis from the pathologist was squamous cell carcinoma, a serious metastatic cancer that has a poor prognosis. I consulted with a veterinary oncologist in Tucson regarding treatment. Her opinion was that Judy was beyond significant help and the best we could hope for was temporary alleviation of some, but not all, of her clinical signs. As difficult as the decision was, we all agreed that euthanasia was indicated. We spread her ashes in one of the big draws where we often hunted quail and enjoyed being with Judy.

I like to think Judy's life and "near death" experiences send us a message, a "moral to the story" if you will. Two times she faced the most dire circumstances that one can imagine. She was staring death in the eye each time and survived both and went on to live a wonderful life. The "take away": no matter how hopeless one's situation and future appear to be, help might be pulling into the driveway right now and in short order your life will change for the better, far better than you ever imagined it could be. Don't give up.

There are so many stories to tell about her

and her occasional "strangeness" that it will take a book to cover them all. For now though, suffice it to say that many years later we have fond memories of her and we talk about her often. The saying "Who Rescued Who?" was very appropriate with Judy in our lives, as she became an important member of our families.